COMMONSENSE GERIATRICS

I dedicate this book to my wife and daughter and a generation of elderly patients who have taught me so much.

COMMONSENSE GERIATRICS

Keith Thompson
*General Practitioner,
Croydon, Surrey*

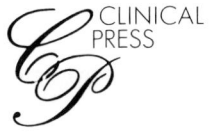

© Clinical Press Limited 1990

All rights reserved. No part of this publication may be reproduced, stored in a retrieval system, or transmitted in any form or by any means, electronic, mechanical, photocopying, recording or otherwise, without the prior permission of the Copyright Owner.

Published by Clinical Press Limited,

Redland Green Farm, Redland Green, Redland, Bristol, BS6 6HF

British Library Cataloguing in Publication Data

Thompson, M. Keith (Malcolm Keith)
   Commonsense Geriatrics
   1. Old persons. Medical care
   I. Title

ISBN 1-85457-007-2

Lasertypeset by Martin Lister Publishing Services, Carnforth, Lancs

Printed in the UK by Butler & Tanner Limited, Frome and London

Contents

Section 1 FIRST PRINCIPLES
Population and population structure	1
World population	1
A measure of health in the UK	1
Old people in the practice	6
Basic facts	6
How many?	7
Mortality	7
Morbidity	8
Chronic conditions	7
Consultation rates	11
General practice	11
Referrals to consultant	13
Hospital	13
Social problems	15
Basic principles	16
Social class factor	16
Sex differences	17
Family	17
Parent–child relationships	17
Grandparenthood	17
Sibling relationship	17
The spouse	17
Family business	18
The future family	18
Past occupation	18
Education	18
Ethnic group	19
Special difficulties	20
Low expectations of health care	20
Self-reporting of illness	20
Third party reports	20
Communication problems	20
Altered surface anatomy	20
Multiple pathology	21
Atypical presentation of disease	21
Undefined normal laboratory values	21
Polypharmacy	21
The borderline functional state of organs	21
Insidious onset of diseases	22
Unexpected recovery	22
Environment	22

The effect of cold	22
The effect of heat	22
Falls	22
Inner city	23
Country	23
High-rise dwellers	23
New town	23
The importance of attitudes in the care of the elderly	24
Special difficulties with older patients	24
Myths and partial truths	24
Communication difficulties	26
Hearing	26
Vision	26
Amnestic difficulties	26
Speech	27
Practice organization	27
Preventive care	27
Screening	28
Notes on setting up a clinic	28
The procedure	28
Evaluation	29
Discussion of points for and against screening	32
The team concept	34
A taxonomy of teams	34
Nuclear	34
Extended	34
Homogeneous	34
Heterogeneous	34
Complex	35
Roles in the care of the elderly	35
Division of labour	36
Recurrent social problems reinforcing medical need for hospital admission	38
The role of the doctor	39
The history	39
The examination	40
The special senses	40
The eyes	41
The ears	42
Upper and lower limbs	43
The spine	45
The chest	46
The heart	47
The neck	48
The alimentary system	49
The rectum	49
Conclusion	50
The investigation	50
The interpretation of test results	51
Normal laboratory values for elderly patients	53

Hospital admission	54
What should be the content of the doctor's letter?	54
Alternatives to admission	55
Be a personal doctor	55
Health education and follow-up	56

Section 2 THE AGEING PROCESS

The ageing process	58
The epidemiology of ageing	58
Genetic aspects of ageing	59
Ageing at cellular level	60
The biology of ageing and the ageing of physiological function	61
Human development and gerontology	63
The energy and reproductive homeostats	64
Changes in appearance and function	69
The eyes	69
Hearing	69
Changes in function	70
Psychological aspects fo ageing	71
Effects of environmental factors and life patterns on life span	74
The influence of obesity	75
The role of exercise in ageing	77
Smoking	79
Stress and accelerated ageing	80

Section 3 COMMON CLINICAL PROBLEMS

Anorexia and nutritional problems	84
Dysphagia	85
Weight loss	86
Points to note in the history	86
Points to notice in the physical examination	88
Investigations	88
Loss of energy and the complaint of fatigue	89
Sleep disorders and insomnia	90
Attitudes to sleep	90
Common causes of sleep disorder	91
Review of the drug list	91
To prescribe or not to prescribe	92
A practical approach to sleep disorders	92
Headache	93
Check list of causes of headache in the elderly	93
Dizzy turns and unsteadiness	94
Labyrinthine and CNS abnormalities	94
Circulatory and metabolic disorders	94
Falling in the elderly	95
Points to remember when examining someone who has fallen	96
Sight and hearing	97
Vision and age changes	97
Ageing and vision	98
Extraocular causes of visual impairment	98

Ocular causes of visual impairment	99
Vascular occlusion	100
Macular degeneration	100
Ageing and hearing loss	100
Dyspnoea on exertion	102
Cardiovascular causes	103
Congestive cardiac failure	104
Diagnosis	105
Blood pressure in old age	107
Guiding principles for treating arterial hypertension	108
Postural hypotension	109
Chest pain	109
Back pain in the elderly	110
The painful hip joint	113
Examination	113
Management	114
Skin irritation	114
Oedema of the lower limbs	116
Management	117
Shakiness and tremor: ageing or disease?	117
Sex problems	119
Some facts	119
Altered bowel function	121
Incontinence	122
The home visit	123
When to refer	124
Management	124
Drug treatment	125
Follow-up	125
Acute confusion	126
Hypothermia	127
Prognosis	130
Hyperthermia	130

Section 4 SPECIALITY ASPECTS

Cardiovascular disease	134
Diseases of the veins	136
Pulmonary embolism	137
Anticoagulants	137
Peripheral arterial disease	137
Cerebrovascular disease	137
Respiratory disease	138
Pneumonia	139
Bacteriology	140
Supportive measures	140
Disorders of the alimentary system	141
The oesophagus	142
Peptic ulcer	142
Gallstones	142
Jaundice	142

Diverticular disease	143
Laxative abuse	143
Faecal incontinence	143
The locomotor system	143
Joint disorders	143
Bone disorders	144
Muscle disorders	145
Endocrine disorders	145
Thyroid disease	145
Diabetes mellitus	146
Obesity	147
The blood	148
Anaemia	148
Iron defficiency anaemia	148
Megaloblastic anaemia	149
Neurological disorders	150
Parkinson's disease	150
Herpes zoster and post-herpetic neuralgia	150
Degenerative neurological disorders	151
Mental disorders	151
Affective disorders	151
Common emotional problems in the elderly	153
Anxiety in the elderly	155
Management of anxiety in the older person	157
Depression	157
Intellectual failure	159
Problems in the diagnosis of dementia	159
Language impairment	160
Mental testing	160
Language function	161
Definition of dementia	161
Managment	162
The future	162
The feet	163

Section 5 SOCIETY, FAMILY AND COMMUNITY

At risk groups	164
Living alone	166
Retirement	168
Bereavement	
Cultural aspects	175
Institutionalization	176
Housing	178

Section 6 USES OF.....

Uses of drugs	182
Factors affecting drug action in the elderly	182
Helpful guidelines in prescribing	183
Practical suggestions	184
Use of the team	185

The team as a whole	185
Team function	186
Formulation of objectives	186
A model	186
Use of the hospital	187
How far is the hospital a community resource?	187
When and what to refer	188
What to say	188
Investigations	189
The day hospital	189
Uses of practice clinics	189
Assessment clinics	189
Clinics for special groups	190
The use of surveillance	190
Use of day centres, community clinics	191
Use of volunteers	191

Section VII THE WHOLE PERSON

The whole person	194
What are the aims of care of the elderly?	194
Who is involved?	195
Levels of care	195
The advantage of a generalist	196
The doctor as the leader of the team	197
Where to care?	197
What does the patient want?	197
The dying patient	198

Index   201

Section 1
First Principles

POPULATION AND POPULATION STRUCTURE

WORLD POPULATION

The expectation of life at birth in developed countries is generally much higher than in countries where random causes of death still occur widely. There are also great disparities when the proportions of elderly, aged 60 or over, in the total population are compared, and this proportion can be around 20%, as in the UK, or as low as 3% in developing countries. World population, estimated by the UN in 1950 to be about 2.5 billion, is projected to be 6.1 billion in the year 2000.

A measure of health in the UK

Table 1.2 is indicative of improvements in health care, health education, and housing and nutrition since the turn of the century. Note that, until 1979, the expectation of life had been lower at birth than at age 1, reflecting the higher mortality rates of earlier years.

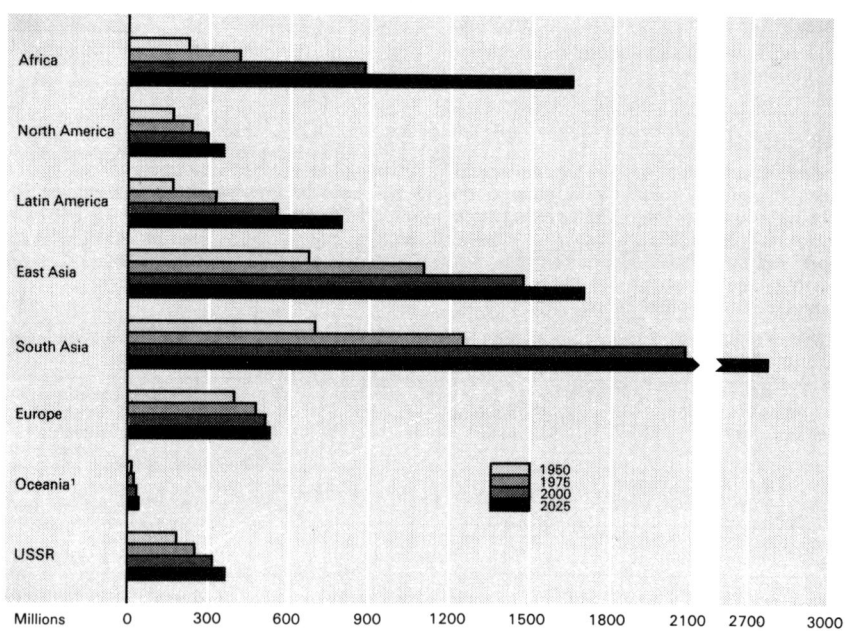

Figure 1.1 World population growth, 1950–2025. Source: World Population Prospects, United Nations

Table 1.1 Population and population structure: selected countries

	Estimates of mid-year population (millions)						Percentage[1] aged		Expectation of life after birth	
	1961	1971	1976	1981	1983	1984	Under 15	60 or over	Males	Females
United Kingdom	52.8	55.6	55.9	56.4	56.4	56.5	21	20	69.8	76.2
Belgium	9.2	9.7	9.8	9.9	9.9	9.9	20	18	68.6	75.1
Denmark	4.6	5.0	5.1	5.1	5.1	5.1	20	20	71.1	77.2
France	46.2	51.2	52.9	54.0	54.6	54.9	22	18	70.1	78.2
Germany (Fed Rep)[2]	56.2	61.3	61.5	61.7	61.4	61.2	18	20	69.9	76.6
Greece	8.4	8.8	9.2	9.7	9.8	9.9	22	17	70.1	73.6
Irish Republic	2.8	3.0	3.2	3.4	3.5	3.5	31	15	68.8	73.5
Italy	49.9	54.0	56.2	57.2	56.8	57.0	22	17	69.7	75.9
Luxembourg	0.3	0.3	0.4	0.4	0.4	0.4	19	18	66.8	72.8
Netherlands	11.6	13.2	13.8	14.2	14.4	14.4	22	16	72.4	79.2
European community[3]	242.0	262.1	268.0	271.9	272.4	272.8	26	15	65.1	72.9
Portugal	8.9	9.0	9.7	9.9	10.0	10.2	27	15	69.7	75.0
Spain	30.6	34.1	36.0	37.6	38.2	38.7	19	22	73.0	79.1
Sweden	7.5	8.1	8.2	8.3	8.3	8.3	25	14	71.4	78.4
Australia	10.5	12.9	13.9	14.9	15.4	15.5	36[5]	13	64.0	74.0
USSR	218.0	245.1	256.7	267.7	272.5	275.0	40	6	51.6	53.8
Egypt	26.6	34.1	37.9	43.5	45.9	—	46	4[6]	48.8	52.2
Tanzania	10.6	13.6	16.4	19.2	20.4	21.1	51	3	51.8	55.3
Zimbabwe	4.0	5.5	6.3	7.4	7.7	8.0	—	—	66.0	68.6
China	671.0	840.0	908.3	1007.8	1039.7	1051.6	39	6	46.4	44.7
India	439.0	551.3	613.3	683.8	732.3	746.7	23	13	73.8	79.1
Japan[4]	94.0	105.7	112.8	117.6	119.3	120.0	23	13	70.2	77.5
Canada	18.3	21.6	23.0	24.2	24.9	25.1	22	16	69.9	77.8
USA	183.8	206.2	215.1	229.8	234.5	236.7	37	6	57.6	61.1
Brazil	71.8	95.2	109.2	121.6	129.7	132.6	43	5	52.6	55.5
Peru	10.3	13.8	15.6	17.8	18.7	19.2				

[1]Latest available year; [2]Includes West Berlin; [3]Includes United Kingdom, Irish Republic, Denmark, and Greece througout
[4]Includes Okinawa; [5]Under 20; [6]65 or over. Source: Government Actuary's Department; Demographic Year Books and Monthly Bulletin of Statistics, United Nations

Table 1.2 Expectation of life from birth and from specific ages

	Males						Females					
	1901	1931	1951	1961	1971	1981	1901	1931	1951	1961	1971	1981
Expectation of life[1]:												
From birth	48.0	58.4	66.2	67.9	68.8	69.8	51.6	62.4	71.2	73.8	75.0	76.2
From age												
1 year	55.0	62.1	67.5	68.6	69.2	69.6	57.4	65.1	72.1	74.2	75.2	76.1
10 years	51.4	55.6	59.1	60.0	60.5	60.8	53.9	58.6	63.6	65.6	66.5	67.2
15 years	46.9	51.1	54.3	55.1	55.6	55.9	49.5	54.0	58.7	60.6	61.6	62.3
20 years	42.7	46.7	49.5	50.4	50.9	51.2	45.2	49.6	53.9	55.7	56.7	57.4
30 years	34.6	38.1	40.2	40.9	41.3	41.6	36.9	41.0	44.4	46.0	47.0	47.6
40 years	26.8	29.5	30.9	31.5	31.9	32.0	29.1	32.4	35.1	36.5	37.3	38.0
45 years	23.2	25.5	26.4	26.9	27.3	27.5	25.3	28.2	30.6	31.9	32.7	33.3
50 years	19.7	21.6	22.2	22.6	23.0	23.1	21.6	24.1	26.2	27.4	28.3	29.0
60 years	13.4	14.4	14.8	15.0	15.3	15.6	14.9	16.4	17.9	19.0	19.8	20.6
65 years	10.8	11.3	11.7	11.9	12.1	12.4	11.9	13.0	14.2	15.1	16.0	16.7
70 years	8.4	8.6	9.0	9.3	9.5	9.5	9.2	10.0	10.9	11.7	12.5	13.2
75 years	6.4	6.4	6.7	7.0	7.3	7.4	7.1	7.4	8.0	8.7	9.4	10.0
80 years	4.9	4.8	4.8	5.2	5.5	5.5	5.4	5.4	5.8	6.3	6.9	7.3

[1]Further numbers of years which a person could expect to live
See Appendix, Part 7: Expectation of life
Source: Government Actuary's Department

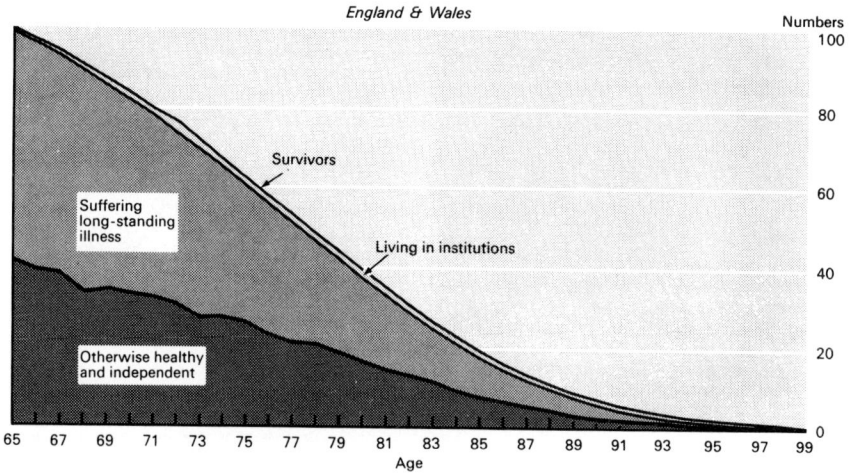

Figure 1.2 Survivors beyond age 65: expectation of life for males, 1981–1983. *Source: World Population Prospects, United Nations*

Despite their differences in life expectations, men and women aged over 65 show similar patterns of health and independence as measured on the Figures 1.2 and 1.3. These tables show the survivors at each year of age from an initial population of 100 people at age 65, and clearly

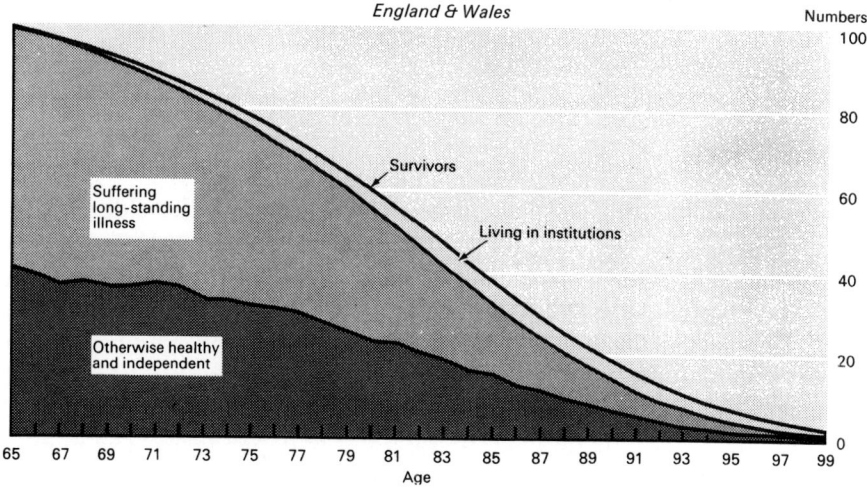

Figure 1.3 Survivors beyond age 65: expectation of life for females, 1981–1983. *Source: World Population Prospects, United Nations*

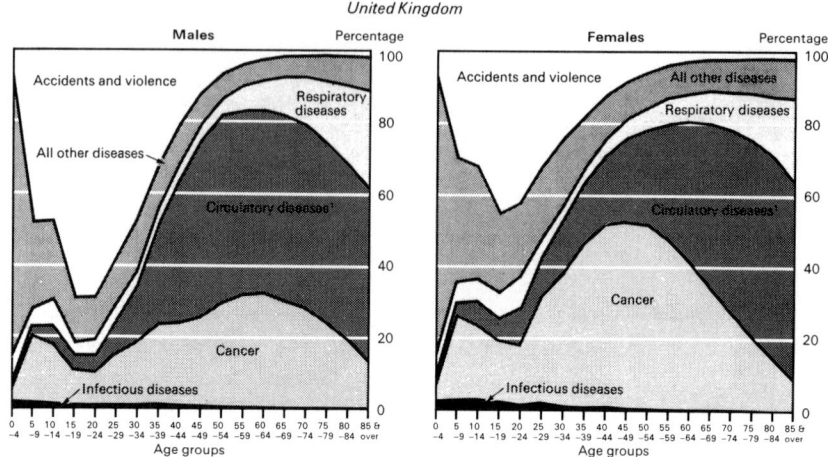

Figure 1.4 Selected causes of death: by sex and age, 1983. *Source: World Population Prospects, United Nations*

show the greater expectation of life for women. For instance, at age 80, 60 of the original 100 women at age 65 are alive; only 40 men survive.

It is also worth considering selected causes of death by sex and age. Figure 1.4 shows that in the UK in 1983 almost half the 659,000 deaths were due to circulatory disorders. Cancer was the next largest cause with proportionately more women dying from this condition than men, up to the age of 70.

OLD PEOPLE IN THE PRACTICE
Basic facts

In an average practice in a typical area, the care of the elderly forms about 45% of a general practitioner's work. On average, 15% of a practice will be over the age of 65, and those over 75 are predominantly female. Health in this age group relates to functional capacity rather than the absence of diseases. Diseases are mainly common conditions which overlap, and are greatly influenced by social and cultural factors. Of those over 70, 20% will be independent, 75% disabled to some extent, but only 5% will be disabled to the point of dependency. The number of elderly in a practice varies greatly from district to district, reaching 45% in some south coast resorts to less than 5% on some new housing estates.

How many?

15% of the population is over 65 years of age. Therefore, in a practice of 2000 patients, there will be 300 elderly distributed as follows:

150 aged 65–74, the young elderly
100 aged 75–84, the old
50 aged 80+, the very old

Future projections indicate some increase in those aged 75–84 and a marked increase in the number of those over 85 by the end of the century.

Mortality

The chief causes of death are:

Circulatory diseases 45%
Cancer 25%
Respiratory diseases 20%
Other diseases 9%
Violence and accidents 1%

Note from Figure 1.4 that the very old are less likely to have cancer, but are more vulnerable to terminal respiratory illness.

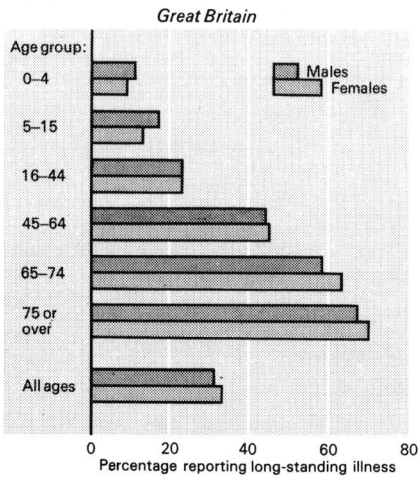

Figure 1.5 Long-standing illness: by age and sex, 1983. *Source: World Population Prospects, United Nations*

Morbidity

Health in the elderly may be assessed in terms of function and of independence. If we consider Figure 1.5, based on the respondents to the General Household Survey, we may see that between 50 and 60% of people over 65 (outside institutions) describe themselves, regardless of age, to be suffering from a long-standing illness. But this reflects a self-perception of illness rather than firm diagnosis, and includes illnesses which do not necessarily restrict activity. Indeed, it may mean that they judge their health in relation to their contemporaries.

Despite differences in life expectation, men and women aged over 65 show similar patterns of health and independence as shown in Table 1.3. Until around the age of 90, approximately 40% of men and women, at each year of age, are classified as otherwise healthy and independent, after which the proportion of survivors thus classified falls rapidly.

Chronic conditions

In the elderly, disorders do not occur singly. Below are listed the main chronic disorders found in my own practice in order of descending incidence:

    Arthritis
    Obesity
    Cardiovascular diseases
    Affective disorders
    Vision and hearing defects
    Skin diseases, ulcers, etc.
    Hypertension
    Mental failure
    Incontinence
    Cancer
    Type II diabetes
    Cerebrovascular disease
    Autoimmune diseases
    Parkinson's and other neurological diseases

We are talking of the over–65s, and a span covering 30 years, so it should be pointed out that some diseases, like diabetes, arise most commonly among the young elderly, and other conditions, like autoimmune disease, is more common in females than males. Other conditions occur

Table 1.3 Survivors beyond age 65[1] – health and independence: by sex, 1981–1983. England & Wales: numbers

	Males				Females			
		In private households				In private households		
	In institutions	Long-standing illness	Otherwise healthy and independent	Total survivors	In Institutions	Long-standing illness	Otherwise healthy and independent	Total survivors
Survivors at age:								
65	0.5	57.5	42.0	100.0	0.4	58.6	41.0	100.0
70	1.5	48.6	33.4	83.5	1.6	53.1	36.5	91.2
75	1.9	34.3	26.2	62.4	3.2	43.0	32.1	78.3
80	2.0	20.9	16.6	39.5	4.5	32.4	23.6	60.5
85	1.8	10.1	7.6	19.5	5.8	17.3	15.3	38.4
90	1.3	0.6	0.7	2.2	3.1	2.3	1.8	7.2

[1]Based on initial populations of 100 men and 100 women at age 64. Expectations of life, health, and independence of the elderly.
Source: Office of Population Censuses and Surveys

Table 1.4 Patients consulting. Rates per 1000 persons at rise. Age-group x College diagnostic code, sex. 1981/2

Males		Reason for consultation	Females	
65–74	75 + over		65–74	75 + over
23.7	24.1	Diabetes mellitus	22.3	22.4
4.9	10.4	Iron deficiency anaemia	10.5	19.1
3.7	5.7	PA	3.6	7.8
2.6	17.8	Senile organic psychotic conditions	4.7	31.4
14.5	14.7	Anxiety state	46.1	34.2
20.5	26.2	Depressive disorder	51.0	44.1
11.5	13.2	Insomnia and other sleep disorders	21.1	18.9
7.0	12.5	Acute stress and adjustment reaction	22.4	18.6
6.4	15.1	Parkinson's disease	6.1	8.6
8.4	10.9	Other diseases of CNS	9.4	9.5
6.2	11.8	Cataract	9.2	18.7
50.5	56.0	Wax in ear canal	31.3	36.7
8.9	10.1	Vertiginous syndromes	13.1	13.0
11.9	21.8	Deafness, various forms	8.3	20.0
11.9	22.4	Acute MI and subacute IHD	11.1	12.8
35.4	31.9	Angina of effort	21.5	22.8
27.0	33.6	Other chronic IHD	16.1	26.0
11.7	21.8	A/F or flutter	9.0	19.1
20.4	67.5	Congestive heart failure	19.2	69.3
10.0	27.4	Left heart failure	5.3	17.7
114.9	75.4	Uncomplicated hypertension, primary and secondary	147.7	96.8
15.3	39.6	Cerebrovascular exc. 437.2	12.5	33.2
11.4	19.4	Transient cerebral ischaemia	6.1	17.7
13.5	15.5	Arterial obstruction and periph. vasc. dis.	7.0	9.5
15.9	15.6	VV of legs with or without ulcer	26.7	21.7
41.1	34.9	Acute non-febrile URI	50.4	44.6
18.6	17.0	Acute febrile URI	18.2	16.5
99.4	127.9	Bronchitis, bronchiolitis, acute	88.5	90.7
37.9	47.5	Chronic bronchitis	13.6	12.3
26.2	31.2	Emphysema, COAD	7.8	7.2
31.5	16.2	Asthma	18.7	12.9
22.7	22.6	Disorders of function of stomach	21.4	20.0
12.9	24.4	Inguinal hernia	0.9	1.8
16.7	33.8	Constipation	14.5	30.3
16.2	30.9	Cystitis and urinary infection	37.9	39.6
17.3	28.4	Benign prostatic hypertrophy	–	–
–	–	Uterovaginal prolapse	10.4	12.3
24.5	22.6	Dermatitis, contact dermatitis, eczema	24.8	18.5
8.3	8.7	Pruritis and related conditions	11.8	12.6
5.4	13.7	Chronic ulcer of skin	7.7	16.3
9.0	11.0	Diseases of skin and s/c tissue	13.2	15.4

Table 1.4 (continued)

Males 65–74	75 + over	Reason for consultation	Females 65–74	75 + over
8.9	9.5	R/A and allied conditions	20.0	18.5
54.9	69.6	O/A and allied conditions	103.7	134.8
30.3	31.9	Back pain, lumbar, thoracic radiation	33.7	34.6
17.6	27.9	Dizziness, giddiness	27.9	37.3
8.5	24.9	Oedema, localized or dependent	20.5	40.2
22.5	23.0	Cough	21.9	21.2
21.7	26.7	Abdominal pain	25.1	27.5
9.0	19.1	Malaise, debility, fatigue, tiredness	19.0	29.2
1.3	23.3	Senescence	2.7	44.0
10.5	11.2	Adv. effect of drug admin. in proper dose	14.2	14.1
13.1	22.7	Bruise contusion or crushing 920–929	23.2	45.6
24.8	34.1	Inoculation v flu	25.4	27.0
34.7	37.3	Letters, forms, certs. and prescription	32.7	39.4

so frequently together, e.g. obesity, hypertension and osteoarthritis of the knees, that they could almost formulate a syndrome.

Consultation rates

General practice

It is interesting to note that the proportion of elderly patients on the list of a general practitioner has little effect on his overall workload. Nor is there evidence of a sharp change in consultation rates at the age of 65 years. The proportion of new consultations (patient initiated) declines steadily with age, so that two-thirds of consultations with the very old are for follow-up care. Recent studies have shown that the overall rate for the elderly was 4.6 consultations per year compared with 2.9 for all patients aged less than 65 years.

As might be imagined, higher proportions of elderly patients are not associated with an increase in the amount of time spent in the surgery, but are associated with more time spent on home visits. The variation between doctors is so considerable in respect of consultation rates per year and the number of home visits per week that no generally applicable statistics can be given. Table 1.5 (Wilkin, D. and Williams, E.I.) is of interest.

Table 1.5 Workload of general practitioners (total n = 178) by the proportion of elderly patients on their lists

% of elderly patients on list	No. of GPs	Mean No. of consultations per pt/year	Mean No. of consultations per elderly patient per year	Mean time spent in surgery per per wk (h)	Mean time spent on home visits per y (min)	Mean time spent with each patient	% of GPs who felt overworked
<10	23	2.8	6.2	15.1	3.3	23	52
10–14	78	3.0	4.6	15.1	4.5	24	59
15–19	68	3.2	4.1	15.0	4.9	27	56
20–25	9	3.1	3.4	13.5	4.2	26	33

From Wilkin, D. and Williams, E.I. (1986). *J R Coll Gen Practit*, 36, 567-70. reproduced with permission

Table 1.6 The pattern of care as a percentage of all consultations in the study population in one year

Age group (years)	No. of consultations	New cases referrals	Home visits referrals	Prescriptions	Lab. tests	Consultant	Other
15–54	44,910	55	5	67	5	7	2
55–64	11,738	39	8	74	3	6	1
65–74	10,224	37	20	80	3	6	2
75+	7,547	33	47	75	2	6	3

From Wilkin, D. and Williams, E.I. (1986). *J R Coll Gen Practit*, 36, 567-70. reproduced with permission

Referrals to consultant

In this study of data collected from 17,771 patients over 65 undertaken by 201 doctors in urban general practices, the mean referral rate to consultants for elderly patients for all doctors was 6% but this concealed large variations between doctors, ranging from rates of more than 10 per 100 consultations to less than two per 100 consultations.

Referrals to consultants declined slightly with age, and none of the general practitioners had access to community hospital beds. For all referrals, more men were referred than women, suggesting that old men may consult with problems perceived by doctors as being more serious.

Surprisingly, it was found that laboratory utilization declined from 5% of all consultations for the 15–54 years age group to 2% for the 75-plus age group.

Hospital

Referral to hospital varies considerably from one GP to another. For instance, it has become unusual to seek admission for acute coronary heart disease for patients over the age of 70, particularly when the home conditions are good. Similarly with stroke illness, some rehabilitate at home, while others believe hospital investigation is always necessary.

> *Female Patient 77 y*
> I was called at 10.30 pm to find 14 members of a large Irish family who lived in adjacent houses all in the street waiting for me. The head man of the family put his head through the car window to say I had got to get her away to the mental hospital because she was a lunatic. He indicated the full moon, and said exactly the same had occurred last full moon. When I asked if I could see my patient, I was asked 'What's the use?". Insisting on the patient's right to see her own doctor, I entered the room and noted a smell of infected urine. Her bedclothes were wet, and there was a tenderness of the right hypochondrium. She had a confusional state. The urological surgeon admitted her next morning, and later a staghorn calculus was removed. She died four years later following a fall on a cliff path in Cornwall.

Table 1.7 Consulations with general practitioners (NHS only): by age and sex, 1983, Great Britain, percentages and numbers

	Age						All ages
	0–4	5–15	16–44	45–64	65–74	75 or over	
General practitioner (GP) consultations							
Percentage of population consulting a GP in the 14 days before interview							
Males	21	10	8	12	18	20	12
Females	20	9	17	15	18	21	16
Average number of GP consultations per person per year							
Males	6.9	2.9	2.3	3.8	5.4	6.6	3.5
Females	6.2	2.8	5.2	4.6	5.9	6.6	4.9
Sample size (=100%)(numbers)							
Males	900	2,258	5,046	2,800	1,060	533	12,597
Females	916	2,067	5,209	3,037	1,419	952	13,600
Ratio of surgery to home consultations							
Males	5.4	7.1	24.2	8.6	3.2	1.2	6.1
Females	4.8	13.4	14.7	5.6	2.5	0.8	5.0

Source: General Household Survey, 1983

Acute admissions will also be decided largely on social grounds, such as degree of family support, and suitable housing. Referrals, on the other hand, depend much more upon a doctor's attitude, and the stage of his education in deciding what he hopes to achieve by further investigation and rehabilitation.

For those over 65 my own figures were:

    Admitted to hospital 15%
    Referred to OPD 25%
    Attend A and E departments 5%

The disease groups causing admission in one year were:

    2 Prostatic surgery
    2 Gynae: prolapse, Ca corpus uteri
    4 Eyes: cataract 3, retinal detachment 1
    8 Cardiac: I.H.D., investigation, pacemaker, etc.
    3 Psychiatric: ECT for depression, acute confusion, dementia Alzheimer's type
    8 Symptoms for investigation: weight loss, chronic diarrhoea, weakness
    5 Respiratory: pulmonary embolism, acute on chronic infection
    1 Haematology: monocytic leukaemia
    2 Trauma: falls, fractured femur
    2 Orthopaedic: hip replacement
    1 Endocrine: virilization resulting from adrenal tumour
    3 GI tract: colectomy, oesophageal dilatation, sigmoidectomy

Social problems

The social component in management of old people is enormous, and its evaluation obligatory. Both admission and discharge rates are modified by factors like housing conditions, neighbourhood support, and by financial and cultural considerations. Relevant to the concept of community care are:

    Housing
    Poverty
    Isolation
    Educational standard
    Faddism
    Continuing employment
    Marital status

Ethnic group
Past occupation
Attitudes to age
Family myths

> I was asked to pay a routine visit to see an 84-year-old man, living alone. I found him to be remarkably independent, and, noting how beautifully clean and orderly were his surroundings, enquired who helped him, for it had been suggested he might need Home Help. Any help was indignantly rejected as he went on to inform me he had served in the Royal Navy, after which he gave me an account of the complete daily routine, worked out strictly according to a programme of bells and watches.

BASIC PRINCIPLES

Social class factor

Living standards in old age are a function of lifelong class position to extent that the elderly poor form an underclass, as well as being persons who would be deprived, whatever their age, by virtue of their class status. Higher social status means, among other things, greater eligibility for inheritance, occupational pensions and greater likelihood of home ownership. An implicit reliance by the state on private pensions reinforces class differences among the elderly. Despite redistributive tendencies of state retirement pensions, it is most likely that low incomes in retirement will follow low status in working life. Those aged over 75 are the poorest group of all, more than half of whom are entitled to supplementary benefit, and a positive correlation exists between advancing age, and diminishing resources. They are the hardest hit by inflation, their living accommodation is likely to be most in need of repair, and their stock of consumer durables is more likely to be inadequate or in poor repair.

As might be expected, one finds, in this group, greater acceptance and enhanced tolerance of the problems of advancing age.

Sex differences

Society makes scant provision for women of pensionable age. The poorest household among the elderly is a one-person household with a widowed woman of lower social class in her mid 70's. Such women are less likely than other elderly persons to have access to a household washing maching, car, refrigerator, telephone and colour TV set.

Family

Every old person is a member of a family, which is often represented photographically because of separation by death or distance. The family history of old people is an important area of enquiry, revealing standards set, conformity and deviation, and the influence on behaviour of children and siblings, and genetic factors.

Parent–child relationships

Old people are warmed by the love of their children. Since this is re-payed on the basis of past relationships, it is wise never to take sides when children are criticized for 'ingratitude'. There is always a reason for this.

Grandparenthood

This is a relationship as much needed by children as by the elderly. I introduced some lonely spinsters to families where there were no grandparents to the advantage of both.

Sibling relationship

More than other relationships, the loss of a sibling is felt as a threat in old age. In estimating health and expectation of life, siblings are of greater value to the GP than are parents who lived through a different generation.

The spouse

The status of males declines, while that of females is raised, in old age because women, as a rule, remain more socially involved, whereas a man's status depends largely on the job he was doing. Men always find resumption of the single state after widowhood more difficult. It is interesting that the indifferent husband is often glorified by his widow after his death.

Family business

This seems to be a dying institution, but, in those rare cases where a family business persists, it provides older people with a wide source of continuing interest.

The future family

The desire to complete child-bearing at an early age, combined with longevity, will increase the number of three- and four-generation families. The trend to more frequent divorce and remarriage, and to cohabitation, sometimes with successive partners, seems set to confuse and weaken the sense of family obligation in the future. Also, with increased longevity, the caring generation may become unable to assume responsibility if they themselves are over 65 years old.

Past occupation

The influence of past occupation on health and behaviour must never be overlooked, particularly in old men. Occupations, which may be several, should be looked at from the point of view of nutrition, activity and exercise, and hazards. Discipline instilled may be missed in retirement, but may also promote order and self care.

Education

We are, at the present time, emerging from the days when most people over 75 left school before the age of 14. Health education, however, was never supplied to the older age group. In each practice, there will be patients who are illiterate or semiliterate. They may be recognized as non-responders to postal surveys, or from an absence of any reading matter within the home. I found some 5% of my older patients had great difficulty with the written word and could be classed as illiterate, men more than women. More particularly, official language relating to pensions, and various allowances, can tax the understanding of many older people and threaten social competence.

It is not uncommon for practitioners to detect, when explaining the meaning of symptoms, that the patient constantly nods in shallow agreement. This may be due to cerebral aspects of the listening process. Too much information, too rapidly given, with the inclusion of a technical word or phrase, may defeat the best of intentions.

Impaired comprehension may be noted for the first time following the death of a spouse or principal helper, or when due to a small focal lesion. Remember that enthusiastic doctors may indulge in jargon fluency and chatty inconsequence!

Ethnic groups

Practitioners are now involved in the management of those from very different cultures. A few important differences will be noted, but this is a study in itself.

Many Asian patients place reliance on self-administered traditional remedies, while habits such as spitting, using handkerchiefs rather than tissues, and hooka smoking, may raise matters for health education. In these cultures, the continued employment of the elderly, and prestige at the head of an extended family needs to be understood and respected. Religious practice may produce difficulties between a male doctor and female patient, or vice versa. Nor should a Christian touch, and so defile, the corpse of a Muslim who has died, and needs to be turned to the east. Other cultural taboos concern – 'low caste' parts of the body such as the anus, genitalia and the feet, cleansing of which is reserved for the left hand only. Naturally, this leads to humiliation, especially for a woman when asked to submit to rectal examination, to insert suppositories, or to be given an enema, all of which are important aspects of geriatric practice.

Finally, there are physical differences to be borne in mind. Negro patients are very unlikely to suffer from osteoporosis, but are very likely to develop arcus senilis in the forties, much earlier than North Europeans. Sikh patients might be very offended if asked about smoking or drinking alcohol, and Hindus would find it difficult, if not impossible, to drink beef tea. Other groups are life-long vegetarians, which may affect such problems as atherosclerotic change and cholesterol levels in later life.

SPECIAL DIFFICULTIES

Low expectations of health care

The young elderly indicate a change from the generation who accepted illness as an inevitable part of the process of ageing.

Self-reporting of illness

Dramatic symptoms, such as pain or vomiting, are reported early, but, despite the utmost availability, many instances occur when symptoms, such as headache, tiredness, weight loss and altered bowel habit are reported late for effective intervention.

It is a good idea to have a special leaflet inviting the old to report any change in health they have noted, and to bring a urine specimen and be prepared for a full examination, for which they should wear clothing that is quickly and easily removed!

Third-party reports

These are often very helpful, but the doctor must be wary of exaggerated reports given out of self interest, and for the avoidance of further involvement.

Communication problems

Because amnestic difficulties are common, and old folk often omit important details of their history, it is often helpful if they write down what they want to report, or if they bring a friend or relative to the consultation for support. I always keep a hearing tube ready for the hard of hearing.

Altered surface anatomy

Most older people develop kyphoscoliosis to some degree. When moderate, this will alter the position of the apex beat and enable a health liver to be palpated. Quite often, an unfolded and calcified aorta will prevent emptying of the left jugular vein, so that both sides of the neck should always be examined. Other features are the finding, on the right side at the base of the neck, of pulsation from the innominate artery brought into prominence at the sterno-clavicular junction by the unfolding of the aorta. Even a redundant loop of sigmoid with diverticulitis may wander across and suggest appendicitis!

Multiple pathology

Finding, say an iron-deficiency anaemia, osteoarthritis, peptic ulcer and cardiac failure, indicates that you have identified several pathologies. But, how do they relate? Is the anaemia contributing to the heart failure? Was that NSAID drug responsible for precipitating excessive salt and water retention, or was the gastric mucosa injured?

Could the patient have purchased salicylate preparations direct from the pharmacist?

Atypical presentation of diseases

Perhaps two-thirds of myocardial infarctions are 'silent' – so it may present with mental confusion. The creps at the bases may not be due to pneumonia, but simply to partial lower-lobe collapse due to kyphosis. In any case, the leucocyte count is no help, and the ESR is often elevated in old people for no apparent reason.

Undefined normal laboratory values

The ranges for serum urate have recently been made more liberal. What about blood sugar? If the normal criteria for younger age groups were applied to the elderly, then many elderly would be labelled as diabetics. Old women have higher serum calcium levels, and so on.

Polypharmacy

This can easily develop if a patient is attending several clinics. There is a trend towards purchasing drugs, formerly prescribed only by doctors, from the chemist. The system of repeat prescriptions is difficult to supervise regularly.

The borderline functional state of organs

Cardiac reserve is reduced, the capacity of the urinary bladder is reduced and kidney function is often marginally impaired. Therefore, prescribing needs care which is not thought of in younger people.

Insidious onset of diseases

Thyrotoxicosis and infective endocarditis are examples of the many diseases which have atypical or insidious modes of onset in the elderly. Others, such as Paget's disease and type II diabetes, are often discovered when routine tests are performed.

Unexpected recovery

There is the occasional patient who appears to be going downhill, either requiring lengthy investigation or waiting for hospital admission, then mysteriously recovers untreated during the time interval.

ENVIRONMENT

The effect of cold

Death rates increase in proportion to the duration of temperature change, irrespective of sex. The association of death rates with temperature is much stronger in the old, reaching a peak of association in 7–10 days from autonomic control failure leading to humoral factors involved in clotting and haemolysis. The time relation is as short as 1–2 days for myocardial infarction, 3–4 days for strokes, and about one week for pneumonia and bronchitis.

The effect of heat

Temperatures maintained above 24 °C for more than 48 h result in increased death rates from cerebrovascular accident and coronary heart disease in people over the age of 70. This was noted particularly in Athens in July 1987. Declining efficiency of the exocrine sweat glands prevents sweating in some two-thirds of elderly females, who may be advised to increase fluid intake of cool fluids, have frequent showers and avoid physical exercise.

Falls

There is a marked seasonal variation in deaths from falls, most occurring in winter. These rates are highest in Scotland and lowest in the south of England, suggesting factors relating to vitamin D formation and bone density.

Inner city

Noise, traffic, pollution, anonymity, street crime, the trend away from small shops to supermarket shopping, overstretched services.

Country

Loneliness, poor bus services, villages changing from communities to commuter areas or antique shop parades, driving out local shops and requiring villagers to travel further for essential provisions.

High-rise dwellers

Isolation on a landing, vandalism of lifts, warehousing in areas away from services.

New town

Separation of residence from sons and daughters in districts often thought to be featureless.

REFERENCES

Bromley, DB. (ed) (1984). Gerontology: Social and Behavioural Perspectives. (London: Croon Helm)

HMSO (1986). Health & Personal Social Services Statistics for England

Qureshi, B. (1986). Management of ethnic Asian patients in general practice. *The Medical Annual*, Gray, DP. (ed) p.155–165 (Bristol: Wright)

HMSO (1986). Social Trends 16

Wilkin, D and Williams, EI. (1986). Patterns of care for the elderly in General Practice. *J R Coll Gen Practit*, 36, 567–570

THE IMPORTANCE OF ATTITUDES IN THE CARE OF THE ELDERLY

Here we are concerned with statements of attitude (which contain an evaluative component) and statements of belief (which are factual). If we consider attitudes, it does not follow that holding a low opinion of old age as a state to be experienced determines the opinion one will have of old people themselves. This can be elaborated to distinguish three areas: attitudes towards the PERSON, i.e. old people as people, attitudes towards the PROCESS, i.e. the process of growing old, and atttitudes towards the STATE, i.e. the state of old age, or being old. This scheme may be refined to allow for attitudes in each of these areas to be relevant either to SELF or to the OTHER. A young doctor, for instance, may feel certain behaviour, such as being apathetic or selfish, or repeating oneself, to be more acceptable in the 60–80 age group than in his own age group. He might thus evaluate certain behaviours of older people as seldom their own fault. This might then be taken to imply that it would be easier to counsel old people on how to modify their ways than to attempt to alter the values of younger people who work with them! It is fundamental, therefore, to examine one's attitude in relation to age, sex and personal experience. Thus, the attitude of a young doctor, who has been concentrating on scientific and medical studies since school days, and who encounters old people for the first time on hospital wards, could be expected to be more pessimistic than that of one from a family with active older members. Also, he may be influenced differently by a practice which conducts a programme of preventive care than he would by one plagued by crises involving old patients that might have been foreseen and prevented. Junior hospital doctors have sometimes expressed their attitudes by referring to old patients as 'dross' or 'old crumbles' without troubling to enquire if they originate from practices that provide continuity of care rather than those alerted merely by social disruption.

SPECIAL DIFFICULTIES WITH OLDER PATIENTS

Myths and partial truths

These are numerous and still widely held, and even shared by some practitioners. For instance, the term 'geriatric' should not be used in general practice, for it has been shown that such a term is used for those in whom illness is advanced, financial status low, and where prospect of a return to home is poor. Other patients of the same age are sent to acute medical wards. Patients are best referred to as, for example, an 82-year-old man recently bereaved and depressed with prostatic hypertrophy thought to be benign, but showing early signs of intellectual impairment; or a 76-year-old woman with type II diabetes, marked obesity and hypertension, now having visual difficulty due to cataract.

The appearance of symptoms, such as unusual nervousness, irritability, depression, unaccountable outbursts of anger, personality change, apathy or withdrawal, are frequently considered par for the course of old age, but would be considered clear indications for psychotherapy in the young. Behavioural characteristics may be due to physical factors, but are often indicators of difficulty in social adjustment.

For several generations, old people have been regarded as asexual beings, simply because they have never been asked about their sexual activities, although admittedly opportunities for meeting partners are reduced.

Other common false beliefs are that old people are no longer capable of work, that they cannot go on learning, and that their development has ceased. Above all, although mental failure is more common in the old, there is a tendency to consider all old people as being somehow intellectually inferior.

It is often difficult for younger people to see the elderly as an asset. So often, particularly in practice, they are seen as a 'burden' but one has only to look at the parts played by elderly people in the theatre and other arts, politics, philosophy, religion and law to see this view is false.

False beliefs are often entertained by elderly people who have adapted poorly. Many believe that, because they are old, they must, *ipso facto*, be ill. Others, trying to make the best of things, over react by making ridiculous claims for themselves, particularly in relation to the young. Females often complain that age has made them ugly, failing to observe that, with care of appearance, beauty will persist into late life of an impressive kind, as depicted by great artists such as Rodin and Rembrandt van Rijn.

The importance of these and other false notions to the GP are that they will affect the transactional analysis in consultation. Old people are often expert at playing games, manipulating the situation by role play, attention seeking and the exploitation of social attitudes. An old lady may express gratitude to a male doctor with a kiss on the cheek, a gesture he might avoid in a young patient. The gracious acceptance of such a gesture from someone who is socially deprived is part of the art of medicine, and the maintenance of poise and impartiality will avoid over dependence in these circumstances.

Finally, care needs to be exercised in the evaluation of information provided by third parties, which is often offered out of self interest. Clearly, many of these difficulties and the way to handle them will only be learned by saturation in the phenomena.

Communication difficulties

Hearing

At the beginning of a consultation, or in Reception areas, the primary care team must satisfy themselves that the lines of communication are clear. The usual form of hearing loss, presbyacusis, is always worst when there are noisy surroundings. Raising voices does not help, and may endanger confidentiality. Hearing aids are frequently out of order or maladjusted.

Vision

Hearing and understanding are not the same. Much of what is said is understood by observing facial movements of expression. Hearing is, therefore, largely a cerebral function. You may find yourself bending and shouting into old ladies' ears and be surprised how little is conveyed. Better to have a speaking tube, or even speak into the bell of the stethoscope, in order that your face can be read.

Direction notices in practice premises should not be placed too high for small stooping people to see them.

Amnestic difficulties

Old people often forget what they wanted to tell you. Some bring a friend or use a list to remind them. The strangeness of practice premises, with crowds, noise and rapid movement, are sufficient to throw someone used to a sheltered life off balance. The tension and anxiety thus caused only make it more difficult to remember how to give a good account of oneself.

Speech

Chatty inconsequence, gratuitous redundancy, clipped sentences, and circumlocution frequently occur when received by the 'kind' doctor. These dysphasic aspects may be socially produced, but could result from hemisphere lesions. On the other hand, impairment in comprehension, common enough in younger patients, is more than likely in old people, so that speech must be slow, information clearly given and limited to accord with receptive capacity.

PRACTICE ORGANIZATION

Each practice should have a plan for care of the elderly, who, as a group, show the widest biological and social differences of any other age groups within the practice. The complex problems they often present do not fit comfortably into a short time slot during a busy consultation session. They are also, as a group, heavy consumers of drugs, indicating the need for regular review of repeat prescribing systems.

Preventive care

Each practice should ask itself the following questions:

(1) Can we provide the needs of the elderly population more effectively than at present?
(2) Do we need to take into account to a greater extent the views of elderly people and their relatives concerning the way we:
   (a) schedule our office hours,
   (b) receive 'phone calls, messages and requests,
   (c) keep our records?
(3) Could improvement in efficiency be reflected in providing better care? If so, can we evaluate the services we offer our elderly patients?
(4) How can the links between team members be better activated and extended to include colleagues in other professions?

Preparation for old age should begin as early in life as possible, so that health education should be a function of all consultations, even from early childhood. A clearer idea of functional capacity can be arrived at in middle age, when health education programmes become intensified in order to delay organ failure. A preventive programme will involve all members of the primary health care team in an integration, not only of work, but of recording.

Screening

The value of screening remains debatable. The early programmes, which took place in the 1950s, produced early diagnosis which, it was assumed, allowed treatment to prevent disability advancing, keeping patients out of hospital by providing adequate treatment and rehabilitation. Later work has shown that screening the elderly is expensive in time and money and not productive of unknown serious disease which might be reversed. You can resolve this in your own mind by defining your attitude to what 'care' means. This diagram (Figure 1.6) demonstrates the iceberg phenomenon of those who have presented with symptoms for diagnosis and those who appear healthy without symptoms.

Notes on setting up a clinic

Define the objectives of the clinic, e.g.:

(1) To detect symptomatic and pre-symptomatic illnesses, noting those which are capable of treatment.
(2) To discover, in order to try to remedy, unmet medical and social needs.
(3) To enhance communication between patient and primary health care team members so that they understand each individual's role.

Discuss with partners, who must be convinced of the value of the preventive approach to the care of the elderly.

Other members of the primary care team must be willing and able to organise their day to attend the clinic. This means obtaining agreement from senior officers in various departments.

Arrange a time on a suitable working day with the practice manager.

Decide which age group. I would suggest those aged over 70.

The procedure

The age/sex register is essential to make a roll of those to be sent for, and to record those who have attended and those for recall.

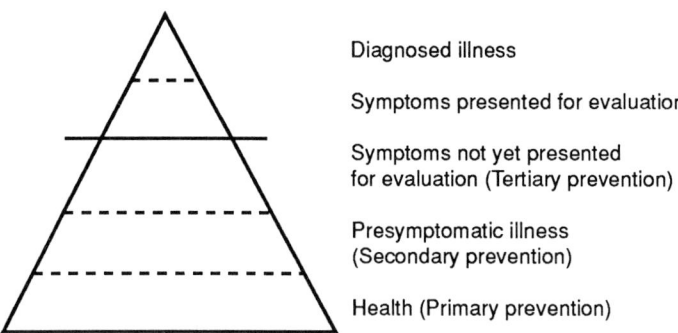

Figure 1.6 The iceberg phenomenon

Decide whether you are going to use a questionnaire and what to call the clinic. We called ours simply the 'over 70's clinic'.

Compose a suitable letter of invitation, of which there are models available at the RCGP.

Define, in advance, the roles of each team member, e.g. the nurse weighs and measures, carries out an audiogram, tests sight with Snellen's chart, tests urine, takes the blood pressure, and checks feet for the need for chiropody.

Assess what facilities you have for blood and biochemistry testing, and the suggestions other colleagues will make, i.e. can use be made of a multichannel autoanalyser, and, if not, what discriminatory tests will you use?

Construct a record card, of which there are again many examples to choose from. None is perfect. Figures 1.7 and 1.8 show the one I have used, both for recording and research purposes.

Evaluation

Evaluation of such programmes should be attempted. Almost all those who have carried out screening programmes consider them to be of value. In certain respects, these are intangible assets, such as improved doctor–patient relationship, quality of life and appreciation of services.

COMMONSENSE GERIATRICS

WOODSIDE HEALTH CENTRE
SCREENING CLINIC FOR THE OVER 70's

Name .... D.O.B ....
Address .... G.P. ....
.... Living alone: YES/NO
.... Principal helper ....
Tel No.

MARRIED	SINGLE	WIDOWED	FAMILY HISTORY
Next of kin:			
....			

SOCIAL AND OCCUPATIONAL HISTORY

Height: .... Weight .... kg
URINE TEST: ....
BLOOD PRESSURE ....../...... ....../...... ....../......
BLOOD SAMPLES
Hb .... WBC .... ESR ....
Hct. .... MCV .... MCBC ....
Blood urea .... TFTs ....
CHEST X-RAY

CHIROPODY	YES	NO

EXAMINATION CARRIED OUT BY DOCTOR

EYES Lids   SKIN
      Vision
      Media   LYMPH NODES
      Fundus
      Glaucoma

HEARING R ....L .... SPINE Kyphosis
NOSE & THROAT ....   Scoliosis
MOUTH ....   Mobility
                                          Pain

NECK Mobility .... LIMBS Clubbing
      Thyroid ....   Weakness
      Vessels ....   Wasting
THORAX Shape ....   Spasticity
Resp. rate   Tremor
Trachea ....   Gait
Lung fields ....   Pulses
             ....   Joints

ABDOMEN   FEET
Contour   Hernia
Scars   Bladder   Oedema
Liver   Aorta
Spleen   Sacrum   Nails
Kidney   P.V.
             P.R.   Skin

SUMMARY

Figure 1.7   (a)   (b)

Psycho-social Report

HOUSEHOLD COMPOSITION   SPEECH
                                         MOOD
HOUSING DATA   MEMORY
    Site   PRAXIS
    Type
    Heating
    Cooking facilities   SYMPTOMS
    W.C.
    Bath   Housing problem   Yes/No   MEDICAL HISTORY   Known diagnosis and current treatment
              Hazard problem   Yes/No

SELF CARE
    Feeding   Drugs taken:
    Washing
    Bathing   ASSESSMENT
    Dressing
    Use of W.C   PROGRAMME
    Shaving
    Hair care Dependent   Yes/No   FOLLOW UP

DOMESTIC CARE   PROGNOSIS
    Cooking
    Housework
    Laundry
    Shopping   Disabled   Yes/No

MOBILITY   Mobility problem

SERVICES   Received   Required
           Health Visitor
           District Nurse
           Home Help
           Meals on Wheels
           Social Worker
           Other

MENTAL TEST SCORE
           Questionnaire   Set test
                              Colours
                              Animals
                              Fruits
                              Towns

Figure 1.8   (a)   (b)

One of the factors contributing to the unpopularity of caring for the elderly has been workload, crisis intervention, etc. Carrying out a full clinical, mental and social assessment does, however, require developed skills and raises the sense of job satisfaction. Patients can be categorized in various ways, e.g.

(1) Independent,
(2) Disabled,
(3) Dependent.

or

(1) Those with definite problems at first test,
(2) Those with a problem expected to cause trouble later,
(3) Those with abnormal findings not expected to be problematic,
(4) Those with no abnormalities.

Evaluation may be made from changes in the Morbidity Index, the nurse's visiting list, etc.

In the first year of my own programme involving the examination of 180 patients, the following important findings were made:
- 77-year-old woman, incontinent of urine, found to have a staghorn calculus, cleared up by ureteronephrectomy
- 3 cases of senile vaginitis
- 2 cases of uterine prolapse, one with a ring pessary not changed for 10y
- 3 type II diabetics
- 2 benign hypertrophy of prostate with major flow-rate reduction
- 3 mental failure cases given trial antidepressants with improvement
- 1 repeated Hb which fell from 11.8G to 7.5G in one month due to PA
- 2 patients blind in one eye due to cataract
- of 17 hearing aids tested, only four were working normally.

That was in 1967. Today, reporting from nurses, social workers and health visitors attached to practice teams has improved, and some of these cases might have been brought to our attention earlier, yet some would have been missed. However, when people are mailed, there will be 'non-responders'. When followed up, the majority will either have moved or died. Of the remainder, we found three main causes: dementia, depression and inability to read. These important findings were dealt with accordingly.

Discussion of points for and against screening

Although extra capitation fees are made for the elderly, the costs involved in running a clinic, though small, might be a deterrent. Against this must be measured benefits in the life of patients, improved doctor–patient relationship, and job satisfaction felt by the team.

Workload appears to be increased, for keeping old people out of hospital requires more supportive services at home. Although some problems might be solved, others are raised. Yet, some evidence exists that workload is ultimately reduced by such a clinic, particularly the unpleasant crises that occur at unsuitable times. Consultation rates do, as might be expected, become less than for practices which rely upon symptom-orientated demand, even in 'favourable' areas.

The main problem, in my experience, lies in the fact that the GP is the longest serving member of the primary health care team, the integrity of which is difficult to retain as other members come and go. It only needs one member's non-cooperation, or poor level of competence, to unbalance the whole scheme.

Increasingly, volunteers are being used to collect health-related data on patients, thus reducing extra work for the primary health care team to a minimum, using charts covering socio-economic problems, problems of disability and basic health questionnaires. They may also be employed, as at Woodside Health Centre, South Norwood, to provide transport, friendly visitors, replacement of hearing-aid batteries, and club facilities.

It has been argued that screening programmes provide little evidence of improvement in the health of the elderly, and proof will always be elusive. Others argue that the principle of confidentiality is at risk by the use of volunteers. Opportunistic case finding has been suggested as preferable, yet it is clear that family doctors do not have time for full assessment of these complex cases in the course of routine clinical care.

References

Barber, J and Wallis, J. (1978). The benefits to an elderly population of notifying geriatric assessment. *J R Coll Gen Practit*, 28, 428–433

Freeman, G, Charlewood, J and Dodds, F. (1978). Screening the aged in general practice. *J R Coll Gen Practit*, 28, 421–425

Freer, CB (1985). Geriatric screening: a reappraisal of preventive strategies in the care of the elderly. *J R Coll Gen Practit*, 35, 288–90

Jones, DA, Victor, CR and Vettner, NJ. (1983). Carers of the elderly in the community. *J R Coll Gen Practit*, 33, 707–710

Pike, LA. (1984). Early intervention in a general practice. In Isaacs, B and Evers, H. (eds) *Innovations in the Care of the Elderly*, Chap4, pp. 25–35. (London: Crook Helm)

Tulloch, A. (1986). Preventive care of the elderly in the community. In Pereira Gray, DJ. (ed) *The Medical Annual*, pp. 45–56. (Bristol: Wright)

THE TEAM CONCEPT

The team concept developed from geriatric medicine in the hospital setting. This suggests than an undercommitment to geriatrics does not dispose a GP to be a good leader of a team. In fact, teamwork across professional boundaries is needed for whole person care.

A taxonomy of teams

It is perhaps desirable to consider the different types of team and how they may apply themselves to varying aspects of general practice work.

Nuclear

Here, there is a close-knit, high-interaction continuum of work relationships, most commonly found between a doctor and receptionist who meet daily. This may also include running a child surveillance clinic with the health visitor, or an antenatal clinic with the midwife.

Extended

Here, the reverse is the case, with infrequent and formalized contacts, such as when a meeting is held to discuss a case of child abuse. There is a need to understand what types of training keep open linkages and pathways between professionals that are relatively infrequently used.

Homogeneous

This is the type that accords with the expectations of many professional workers, namely a team of co-equal individuals, working in a collegial atmosphere, in which specialization by task does not necessarily mean the existence of a skill gradient or hierarchy.

Heterogeneous

This is the type best known to new medical graduates, consisting of an apprenticeship team that is hierarchical, with strong professional and tutelage traditions. The justification for such a team is clearly that there are formally recognized differences in skill, although such differences vary more than perceived variations in the work done.

Complex

This type of team is most suited to care of the elderly where both skills and tasks vary, encompassing multiprofessional and professional/paraprofessional work relationships. A GP, for instance, may find it necessary to carry out a manual removal of faeces urgently on a home visit, and feel able to accept a cup of tea at another, functions which may duplicate those of the nurse and the vicar.

We are concerned here with two factors in care – love and competence. Nurses will find teaching relatives to care in line with professional standard extremely tiring. On the other hand, we cannot teach those trained in a given line of work, to which they apply themselves day after day, to love their charges. It is, however, more practical to train those who have a loving relationship with a given sick person and train them to provide competent care.

The complex team may include members such as ministers of religion (often grossly under-used), newspaper delivery boys, milkmen, street wardens, friendly visitors, and others at various times and in differing circumstances. They can offer advice on preparation to avoid hypothermia, welfare benefits to which they may be entitled, liaison with fuel boards to prevent cut-offs, leisure activities locally available, care strategies, etc. Practical assistance may be offered, i.e. cleaning services after Grant Aid Work, moving house assistance, escort service for shopping and medical visits, liaison with local Social Services Departments, and, after decorating, help with replacing household items.

ROLES IN THE CARE OF THE ELDERLY

Even without a preventive programme, a GP will have got to know most of his elderly patients quite well. He may have cared for the family for more than a generation, observing the changes produced from early middle age to old age. Old people are more static, so that the home is usually known and serial consultations build up to produce a familiar picture.

Of the team members, the receptionist and nurses are well known, especially as 98% of nursing care in the community is concerned with the elderly. Up to the present, health visitors have made a very limited contribution to the care of the elderly, as low as 1.3% in one study embracing 17 practices. This is because they are taught to regard their statutory duty to children under five and to mothers of young children as their

> It was reported to the practice that a 70-year-old female patient had died suddenly in Croydon High Street. The same evening, I paid a visit to the husband in his council house. He introduced me to his widowed sister-in-law who had travelled across from Essex. He told me that I had no need to worry about him, since his wife's sister was going to stay on and look after him. She had a council flat on the other side of London. I realized that, simple as the arrangement sounded, it did create worries in my mind which I did not feel able to solve. The Social Worker attached to us was asked to call next day, and was heavily involved for a week sorting out council regulations concerning such a change, pensions, death grant, removal of furniture, etc.

as their main priority. The potential contribution of health visitors in this field has now been recognized, and there are moves to involve them with old people more in the future.

The social component of pathology in old age is important, but social workers are busy and often only able to deal with problems that are uppermost at the time. Many other matters require attention where old people are ill-informed about their entitlements, or are unaware of the value that could be provided by disability aids.

Despite the accent on the virtues of care in the community by the authorities, there is extremely patchy allocation of needed facilities, such as home helps, mobile meals, chiropody, domiciliary physiotherapy, occupational therapy, day centres and so on. Nevertheless, there is little doubt that a comprehensive system of care for the elderly is beyond economic resources, leading medical and social services with decisions concerning priorities in order to make the best use of resources.

Division of labour

Over a period of several years, I noted various clinical conditions and their responses to treatment and management. These were predominant:

Remediable conditions	*Conditions which can be alleviated*
Primary dietary disease	Deafness
Anaemia	Cervical spondylosis
Depression	Visual defects
Cardiac failure	Arthritis
Faecal impaction	Carcinoma of prostate
Diabetes	Foot defects
Thyroid disorder	Parkinson's disease
Osteomalacia	Diverticulitis
Senile vaginitis	Postural hypotension
Prolapsed uterus	Polymyalgia/cranial arteritis
Hernia	Trigeminal neuralgia
Urinary tract infection	Paget's disease
Prostatic hypertrophy	Chronic chest
	Varicose veins

The main function of the GP in the team was as diagnostician, leading to the need for follow-up and reassessment. Modern practice requires management functions and this is how the division of labour worked:

Doctor	*Nurse*
Cardiovascular disease	Anaemia
Hernia	UTI
Prolapse and gynae	Faecal impaction
Prostatic diseases	Diabetes
Thyroid disorder	Postural hypotension
Osteomalacia	Blood pressure monitoring
Chest disease	Hemiplegia
Visual defects	Carcinomatosis
Parkinson's disease	Gangrene
Varicose veins	Technical nursing
Cervical spondylosis	Training, educating relatives
Giant cell arteritis	
Gangrene	*Social worker/health visitor*
Vertebro/basilar ischaemia	Depression
Diabetes	Diabetes
Emergencies, e.g. acute abdomen	Deafness
	Diverticulitis
	Cerebral failure
	Carcinomatosis

Systematic relief and *Social worker/health visitor*
social support Prevention
Carcinomatosis Early detection
Cerebral failure Identification of need
Hemiplegia Mobilization of resources
Vertebro/basilar ischaemia
Gangrene

The function of the team, in which all disciplines unite, is:

- To reduce pressures of illness and environmental stress
- To boost drive and maintain vigour
- To survey the 'at risk' group continuously
- The step in at the right time
- To cover all patients at risk by selection from the Age/Sex Register.

Recurrent social problems reinforcing medical need for hospital admission

(1) Family strain (27%)
Relatives no longer able to cope with patient
Nearest relative now ill
Relatives cannot afford to stay away from work
The patient is not wanted by his family
(2) Disability disturbing home life (21%)
Patient is incontinent or has dirty habits
Old person now completely bed-fast
The patient has frequent falls
(3) Loneliness (15%)
Patient is always alone without help
Old person alone while family out at work
(4) Mental changes (14%)
Patient has mental confusion
Old person noisy or restless at night
Patient wanders away from home and gets lost
Difficult, temperamental or eccentric old person
(5) Financial problems (11%)
Patient or relatives cannot pay nursing home fees any longer
Landlady reluctant to keep infirm lodger
(6) Other social difficulties (2%)

The role of the doctor

If it is true that the time needed for full assessment is often lacking at times of heavy practice demand, it is nevertheless better to aspire to a systematic approach and to train oneself to achieve it whenever possible. In old people, common conditions are the rule, although atypical presentations may pose more diagnostic difficulty than rare diseases. Even if at some clinical disadvantage technically, compared with hospital colleagues, the home situation provides him with opportunities denied to secondary assessors.

Correct and full diagnosis is of critical importance, recognizing that assessment is often made difficult when impaired cognition and memory are encountered in a person who offers the added physical difficulties of anatomical deformity, voluminous clothing and restricted mobility. This is the field, more than any other, where diagnosis, once arrived at, cedes its importance to considerations of prognosis, and to which sectors effective therapy can be applied.

The history

Whether or not the examination is carried out in the patient's home, there is little doubt that the history is best obtained in a patient's familiar surroundings. There one may grasp more of the patient's life, character, past health, occupation and interests, in order to construct some pictures of what he or she was like in health. Photographs, both of patient and family, taken in earlier days, are often helpful for comparative purposes, and a study of the surroundings is clearly important, providing not only talking points, but stimulation for the patient to respond to questions about events during a heyday, such as a man's army or sporting career, or the time when a woman was the centre of her family.

Full allowance must be made for failing mental powers, and socially conditioned attitudes, such as hostility or loquacity. Apparently irrelevant talk provides the discerning physician with information about spontaneous thought content, mood and preoccupations, and should not at first be discouraged. Indeed, non-aphasic language disturbance, such as gratuitous redundancy and perseveration of ideas, may alert the doctor to hemisphere dysfunction. Similarly, much may be learned by response to questions which show a deficiency of ideas, in short, stereotyped sentences.

The patient should always be addressed by his or her proper name to reinforce the sense of personal identity which may have been eroded through loneliness or depression, or by prolonged use of impersonal terms of address by friends or neighbours, such as 'Ma' or 'old fellow'.

Attempts to hurry the patient beyond his own tempo are self-defeating, and lead to confusion which may be indicated by inappropriate motor responses, such as scratching the head, developing a cough, or losing temper. It is well known that elderly people may vary from day to day in mental performance, and a better result may be obtained at a second consultation. One must also beware following the patient in a tendency to attribute the onset of illness to a particular event, such as a fall or a bereavement, for the onset of disease in old age tends to be insidious rather than precipitate.

Symptoms in the elderly are often described in terms of lost function, such as inability to climb the stairs, rather than as sensations.

The history must establish a time scale on which to place the earliest presenting symptoms, and forge the first link of a chain of events leading up to the present. The interviewer should try to arrange to sit facing the patient so that his face is in a good light and on the same level as that of the patient. The presence of a third party is often welcome in a supporting role by verifying the statements made, but they should not be permitted to take over the interview, but be disciplined to providing information that is supplementary as far as possible.

THE EXAMINATION

This should be carried out with due regard to the patient's ability to co-operate, so that it is not always possible to follow the sequence of physical examination taught at medical school or to match its perfection. Intelligent modifications must be made in accordance with the situations encountered. For instance, it is preferable to listen to the lung bases through a nightshirt than to provoke respiratory distress by making the patient struggle to remove it.

The special senses

It is reasonable to begin the examination by testing the special senses of sight and hearing, as well as the patient's intellectual state, because the efficient conduct of the examination and the interpretation of the findings will depend largely on the integrity of the patient's perceptual

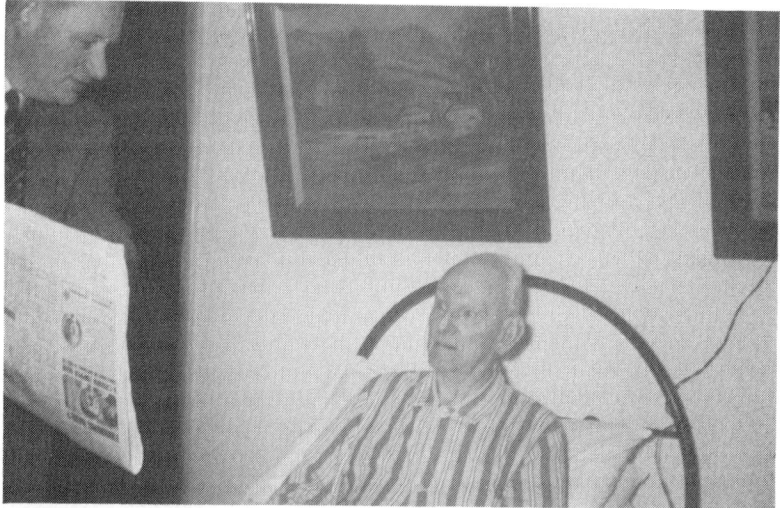

Figure 1.9 Photograph of patient reading paper held at a distance

apparatus. In other words, the lines of communication must be clear. Much can be learned at the bedside without complicated methods of testing, and, here, the widespread habit of newspaper reading in the country is advantageous in that suitable material, printed in letters both large and small, can usually be found lying to hand in most homes (Figure 1.9).

By asking the patient, without gesture, to pick up the paper and read a passage aloud one sets in train a process rich in opportunities for clinical assessment of hearing, language function, praxis and co-ordination, the presence of senile or intention tremor, visual acuity, articulation and vocal quality. A short discussion on the material read will give some indication of short-term memory function and comprehension.

The eyes

Inspection begins with the lids to exclude ectropion or entropion. Conjugate eye movements may reveal nystagmus but it is not uncommon to find, in extreme deviation, irregular eye movements of no pathological significance; or that the full range of upward movement is restricted as a sign of general weakness or, in the absence of raised intracranial pressure, some compromise of the cerebral blood flow. The reaction of the pupils to light and accommodation are often absent in advanced age, or they may show abnormalities due to ocular hypertension, cataract,

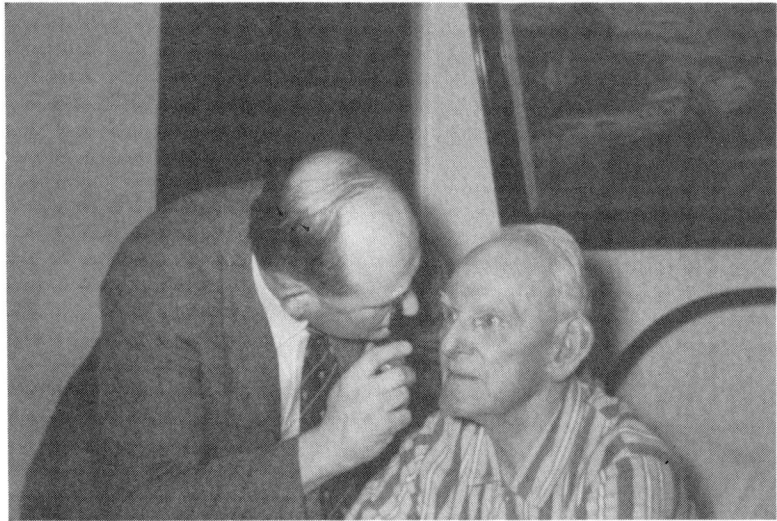

Figure 1.10 Inspection of the anterior part of the eye with the ophthalmoscope

or other intraocular disease. Cataract must be diagnosed by ophthalmoscopic examination (using the 12+ lens) and not assumed to be present if a grey reflex is seen on direct inspection, for this is commonly due to altered refraction of light due to the increased optical density that arises in late age (Figure 1.10).

It must be admitted that the examination of the fundus is often difficult because of opacity of the media, wandering attention of the patient, and the danger of using mydriatic drops to dilate the small pupil. In fact, it is often more valuable to be able to catch sight of normal healthy retinal vessels than to persist in looking for the varying degrees of narrowing and tortuosity. Pathological changes should lead to a request for specialist examination.

The ears

Make sure the auditory canals are free from hard wax. Soft wax is of no importance and no impediment to hearing. Simple tests of hearing are sufficient and carried out by asking the patient to repeat words at varying distances, at first with the normal, and then with the whispered, voice. I must confess I have found this preferable to the use of the audiometer. If a hearing aid is worn, it should be inspected (see Figure 1.11), as, in a proportion of cases, these aids are found to be defective

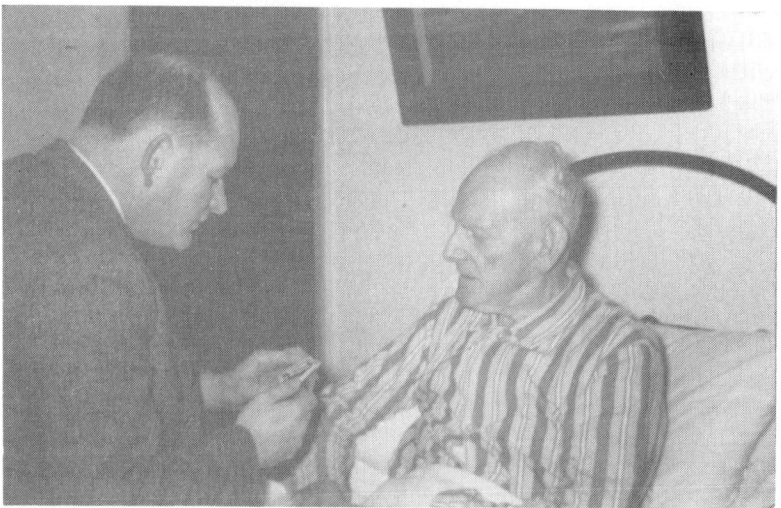

Figure 1.11 Inspecting a hearing aid is an integral part of the physical examination

or incorrectly used. Remember, incidentally, to examine any prosthesis. How often spectacles are covered with grease, preventing clear vision, and artificial limbs are sometimes kept in the cupboard, to be produced only for the doctor's visit!

Upper and lower limbs

Attention is next directed to the upper limbs (Figure 1.12) for signs of wasting, spasticity, rigidity of the Parkinsonian type, flaccidity, or tremor, being careful to exclude that paratonic type of rigidity occasionally met with in old people as a defensive reaction, and which appears immediately when the limb is grasped and resists all efforts at persuasion to relax. The radial pulse is felt, and visible brachial pulsation looked for lateral to the medial epicondyle, after which the hand is carefully inspected.

In the lower limbs, adductor spasm is noted if, when one limb is adducted, the other follows it across the bed. The skin temperature is felt with the dorsal aspect of the fingers, and the feet inspected for colour changes, oedema, digital health, the state of the nails, callosities, and the speed of capilary flow back into the white zone produced by pressure on the pad of the great toe (Figure 1.13). Reflexes are tested in the usual way, but it is as well to realize that anomalies may be

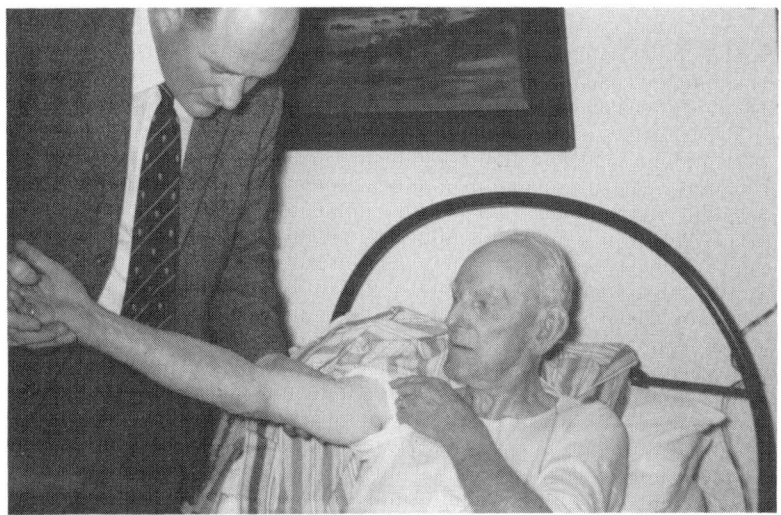

Figure 1.12 Inspecting the upper limb

produced by local disease, so that the plantar response may be mechanically reduced, or even abolished, by hallux rigidus or valgus.

Indeed, as age advances, the tendon reflexes, such as the abdominals, are rarely present in the lower quadrants over the age of 75 years. Sensory testing is seldom successfully carried out, not only because it

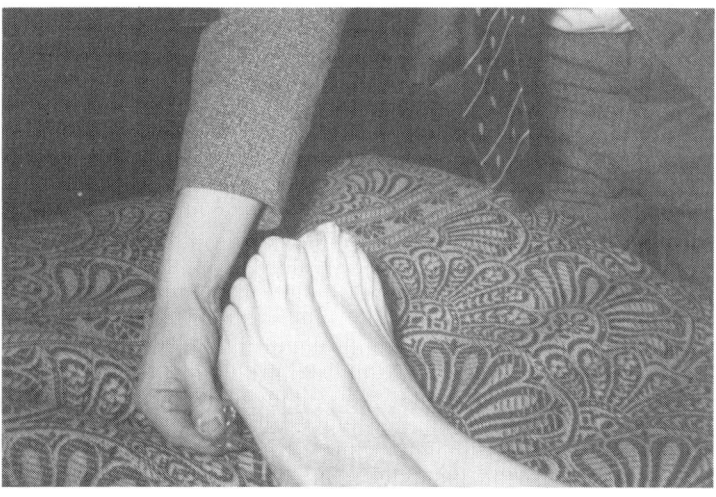

Figure 1.13 Local conditions may produce anomalies of the planter response

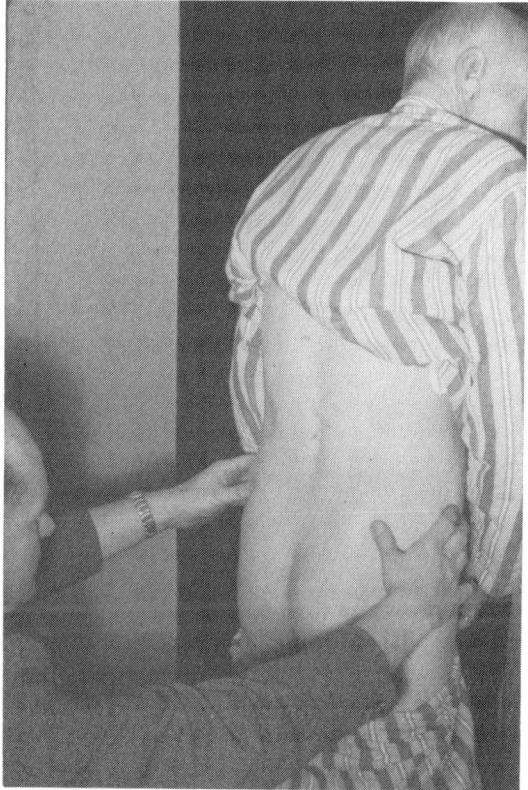

Figure 1.14 Examining the lower spine and looking for pelvic tilt

depends upon patient response, but patchy losses of sensation are often present without necessarily signifying ill health. Vibration sense is very commonly absent below the mid-dorsal region of the spine and in the lower limbs, due to degeneration of the posterior columns.

It is worth mentioning here that, at the same time, primitive reflexes may emerge, such as the pout, palmomental, and nuchocephalic.

The spine

Since old people often sit forward in an almost defensive attitude, the patient can now be asked to stand out of bed at this point so that the spine can be examined for curvatures or pelvic tilt (Figure 1.14).

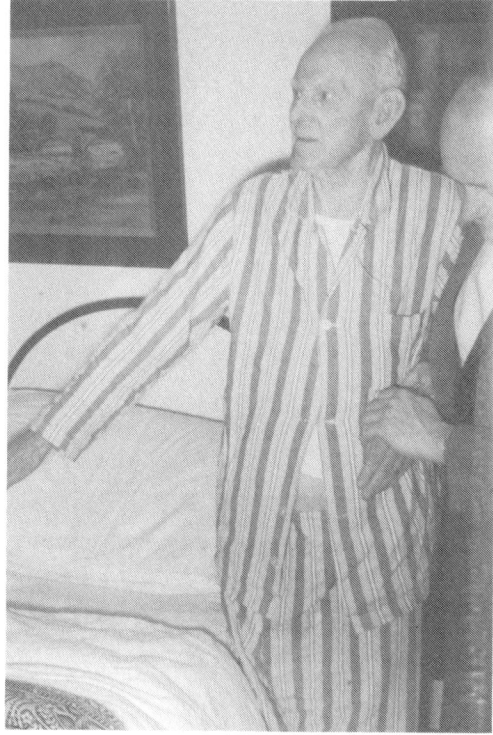

Figure 1.15 Taking the patient on a walk round the bed observing his gait

An opportunity occurs also for testing the strength of the quadriceps while they resist gravity, and note can be made of the presence of contractures, such as flexion deformity of the knee joint. After this, I like to take the patient for a walk around the bed in order to observe his gait (Figure 1.15).

In small rooms, this is difficult, but, even here, one can ask the patient to walk along a line in heel-to-toe fashion in order to look for circumduction of the leg at the hip, for scissor gait or *marche a petits pas*.

The chest

For examination of the chest, the patient is asked to sit on the edge of the bed. On inspection, it is usual to see some degree of deformity of the thoracic cage and it is important to note this because, where kyphoscoliotic changes are marked, they may be sufficient to cause real or apparent displacement or organs in relation to it, so that erroneous conclusions may be drawn. Thus, it may be possible to feel the edge of a healthy normal-sized liver below the costal margin, while narrowing of the anterio–posterior thoracic dimension may displace the heart laterally, allowing the impulse of the apex to be felt outside the midclavicular line and so suggest to the unwary the presence of a cardiomegaly. In the female, the breasts are palpated as she sits on the bed, and, if asked to stand so that inspection can be carried out from in front, it is not unusual to see the transverse sulcus across the upper abdomen, indicating osteoporotic change in the spine. One can then examine the heart and lungs in the usual way.

The heart

Arrythmias are of common occurrence in old age. The dominant arrythmia is atrial fibrillation, commonly associated with acute infections, surgical operations, cardiac ischaemia, pulmonary embolism, thyrotoxicosis, and heart failure, especially when associated with rheumatic heart disease, now seen less commonly. The presence of altered rhythm will direct the examiner to look for peripheral oedema, which, in bedridden patients, may be localized to the sacral region. The incidence of ischaemic heart disease rises with age but the diagnosis may be rendered difficult due to reduced, or absent, sensation of cardiac pain in old age. Special note must therefore be made of the sudden development of heart failure, gallop rhythm or elevation of the venous pressure.

Abnormalities of the aortic valve are common over the age of 70, and ejection murmurs occur as a result of aortic valvular sclerosis, or from true aortic stenosis with definite obstruction to outflow. The conduction of such murmurs should always be followed towards the neck. Though often asymptomatic, aortic stenosis may cause dyspnoea, angina or syncopal attacks, and obstruction to flow, manifesting itself as an anacrotic pulse, reversed splitting of the second sound and left ventricular hypertrophy. It is important, therefore, to attempt to distinguish this condition from valvular sclerosis, where the ejection murmur is less loud and harsh, for, in the absence of symptoms, aortic stenosis carries a good prognosis. It is important also to bear in mind the possibility of infective endocarditis because the classical manifestations are usually lacking in older patients, who may present with mental symptoms or progressive renal failure. Furthermore, the finding of splinter haemorrhages is unreliable, since similar changes appear in the nails of those bearing heavily on walking aids. It is better to observe them in the conjunctivae. The incidence of pulmonary embolism rises sharply in the later decades, in association with cardiac failure, obesity, fractured femur and chronic disease of the leg veins. The classical presentation with pleurisy and haemoptysis is less common, and the clinical features are often varied, with arrythmias accompanied by tachypnoea and minimal signs in the calves. The blood pressure may be taken at this point, noting any drop more than 15 mmHg between the sitting and standing position.

The neck

The neck is important, largely because the four main blood vessels supplying the brain pass through it. The patient is returned to bed in a reclining position in a good light for inspection of the thyroid and the neck veins. The patient may also be asked to demonstrate the degree of retained movement in the cervical joints.

First, it is important to get rid of anomalies. One may note, for instance, two of these. During deep inspiration, the pressure in the two jugular systems equalizes so it is important to observe the venous pressure during this phase. However, delay in emptying the left external jugular may be observed, suggesting a diagnosis of cardiac failure unless care is taken to examine both sides. This unilateral failure to empty is due to delay caused by an unfolded aorta. Also, in hypertensive females particularly, a pulsatile swelling may be observed at the right sternoclavicular region due to unfolding of an arteriosclerotic aorta bringing the innominate artery pulsation into prominence, which has occasionally been mistaken for an aortic aneurysm.

Because of their importance to the cerebral circulation, particular attention is paid to the quality of pulsation in each carotid artery, and gentle pressure may be applied to each artery in turn deep to the anterior border of the sternomastoid. Arterial bruits deriving from carotid stenosis become louder distally because they usually originate at the carotid sinus where the vessel dilates at the proximal part of the internal carotid artery at the level of the upper border of the thyroid cartilage. A bruit transmitted from the heart, however, will be heard over both carotids and will tend to diminish gradually as the stethoscope is moved up the neck.

The alimentary system

Careful examination of the mouth, with inspection of the tongue and teeth is important. Many old mouths are neglected and edentulous. Many also date from the days of the 'plastic mouth' in the 20's and 30's, so that, if false teeth are worn they should be examined *in situ* for their usefulness.

While examining the abdomen, it helps to engage the patient in conversation in order to encourage relaxation. You can then be inspecting the abdominal contours and take visual note of lax skin, scars, herniae, or the presence of visible masses or peristalsis. Small scars will bring to mind the possibility of a pacemaker. The pulsation of the abdominal aorta, prominent in thin people, is a reminder that aneurysmal dilatation may be found at this point.

The rectum

Firm masses felt in the left iliac fossa are often puzzling, and their identity is confirmed when they are indented by the examining finger *per rectum*, pressing laterally into the sigmoid. The presence of an impacted faecal mass in the rectum, with distension of the lax sphincter, is not an uncommon cause of spurious diarrhoea, especially where the patient has been dehydrated over a long period by the unwisely prolonged use of diuretic drugs.

The prostate gland in elderly men is often enlarged, and, in many instances, biochemical tests are required before its benign character can be assured. It is no longer maintained that the acid phosphatase level must not be assessed until at least 48 hours have elapsed after digital examination of the prostate. It is wise to look at the abdomen at this point to see if there is distension of the bladder. If possible, the patient should be asked to pass urine, and one may be fortunate enough to be able to observe the act of micturition for signs of hesitancy, interruption and *vis a tergo*. After emptying the bladder, it is advisable to perform a bimanual examination on a male patient for two reasons: firstly, middle lobe enlargement can only be felt in this way, and, secondly, a rough idea of the amount of residual urine present may be gained by feeling distension of the retroprostatic pouch.

Conclusion

The examination then is directed towards vulnerable areas and practice in the routine sequence will shorten the total time taken.

THE INVESTIGATION

Accurate diagnosis must be the cornerstone of effective medical care of the elderly, so it is no longer assumed that investigation is a wasted effort now that it is clear that many diseases can be treated as effectively as in the young.

Investigations have, as their object, the making of an accurate diagnosis so that an acceptable form of treatment can be recommended. Failing this, they may serve to provide a firmer basis for the prognosis. However, old people are vulnerable to the risks of certain technical investigations and taxing procedures must be carefully weighed in relation to their material value to the patient. It is also as well to remember that some patients undergo extensive investigation until it is realized that depression, the great imitator, is the primary rather than a secondary reaction to feeling ill.

It is also worth remembering that most investigations in general practice are undertaken to determine the nature of symptoms of relatively slow evolution due to conditions which are common, rather than rare, but which may present in an atypical fashion. Also, whereas it is sometimes said that 50% of cases can be diagnosed on the history alone, it is a bold claim to make in the challenging conditions of geriatric practice.

Investigation then should be carried out with the minimum of inconvenience to the patient. Increasingly, despite the fact that there is a certain pride in ordering discretionary tests to confirm the clinical findings, some practitioners now have access to the autoanalyzer, and may use screening methods searching for information without a definite clinical indication. In the elderly, there is a good case for obtaining a laboratory profile which can be carried out cheaply on a small blood sample by multichannel analysis, but it has been suggested that it is essential that the clinician should master the screening as well as the discretionary methods of evaluating test results.

To avoid sources of error, specimens should be taken at the same time of day, in the recumbent position, with care taken to avoid excessive cuffing during venepuncture. The most useful tests in the elderly are:

Full blood count
ESR
Urinanalysis
Serum sodium
Serum potassium
Serum albumin
Serum globulin
Serum calcium
Serum inorganic phosphate
Serum alkaline phosphatase
Serum T4 and T3 uptake
Blood urea
Blood glucose and glycosylated Hb
[random blood glucose taken midmorning]
Serum bilirubin
Serum aspartate transaminase

Results may be misleading for various reasons, e.g. dehydration, protein binding phenomena, etc.

If a test gives an uncertain result, it is better to use an alternative test rather than repeat one in which the second result may not be viewed with certainty. Being too disease-orientated may be less helpful than attempting to promote health, and much of the GP's time must be spent trying to help the elderly to live with their handicaps, rather than trying to correct every deviation from healthy norms.

The interpretation of test results

Looking for anaemia clinically belongs to the field of the amateur. It can only be detected by Hb estimation and film examination. Anaemia is always pathological and is found in 30% of hospital admissions. It is usually a secondary phenomenon, most often due to gastrointestinal bleeding. Whatever type of deficiency is suggested by the blood picture, the serum levels of the three main haematinics should be sought.

The chest X-ray in the elderly is largely requested to exclude malignant disease, pulmonary emboli, and to estimate heart size. The ECG offers the only way to sort out causes of arrhythmias, and a normal ECG almost certainly rules out heart failure, so that it is an essential aid to prescribing.

The wide range of ESR in the elderly diminishes its value as a diagnostic aid, although grossly elevated levels (sometimes found for no apparent reason) are useful indicators of autoimmune diseases. Serum albumin and globulin provide more useful information in the investigation of the elderly.

The blood urea is generally a more useful test than the serum creatinine which needs to be corrected for body weight. Abnormally low levels may be due to fluid overload, low dietary protein intake, or the syndrome of inappropriate antidiuretic hormone secretion (SIADH). Maximum specific gravity of urine has decreased to 1.024 by 80 years of age. The finding of infected urine is common in asymptomatic people, and attempts to eradicate it are followed by a high rate of failure. Best to note that, in the aged, it runs a relatively benign course, and advice on complete bladder emptying is more important than antibiotics.

Uric acid levels can only be reliably interpreted when it has been established that there is good renal function.

Serum levels are not a true indication of the intracellular potassium ion. Delay in sending specimens also allows potassium leakage from red cells. Diuretics are a less important source of potassium loss than are corticosteroids. It is worth remembering that the correction of anaemia rapidly increases potassium demand by newly formed cells.

Glycosuria almost certainly indicates diabetes, but only about half those with significant hyperglycaemia have glycosuria because the renal threshold for glucose is often raised in the elderly. The most practical test is a random blood sugar, best carried out midmorning.

Albumin values tend to mirror the severity of illness, and low values are indicators of poor prognosis. They should be included in a routine profile, not so much for themselves, but because they influence estimations of the substances they transport, for example, T4, cortisol and calcium. Whereas albumin values lower with age, globulin values increase with age and are a little higher in the sick.

Although used in the diagnosis of metabolic bone disease, calcium, phosphate and alkaline phosphatase estimations are more often altered by other causes in the elderly, such as dehydration and treatment with corticosteroids. Normal calcium levels tend to fall with age in men, but rise in women, the reverse being the case, of course, in phosphate values.

Since unrecognized hypothyroidism has been detected in 2% of hospital admissions and unsuspected hyperthyroidism in 1%, there is a strong case for estimating thyroid function routinely in the elderly. Serum T4 has proved to be a practical test in clinical use and results indicative of hypothyroidism should be supported by an estimate of TSH.

Normal laboratory values for elderly patients

Haematological indices
Haemoglobin (men)	11.8–16.8 g/dl
Haemoglobin (women)	11.1–15.5 g/dl
MCV	82–96 fl
HCT (men)	42–54%
HCT (women)	36–48%
WCC	3.1–8.9 x 10^9/L
Serum iron	8.8–30.3 μmol/L
TIBC	38.3–87.0 μmol/L

Biochemical indices
Serum albumin	33–49 g/L
Serum globulin	33–49 g/L
Sodium	135–146 mmol/L
Potassium	3.6–5.2 mmol/L
Chloride	97–108 mmol/L
Bicarbonate	20–31 mmol/L
Urea	3.9–9.9 mmol/L
Calcium (men)	2.19–2.59 mmol/L
Calcium (women)	2.18–2.68 mmol/L
Phosphate (men)	0.66–1.27 mmol/L
Phosphate (women)	0.94–1.56 mmol/L
Alkaline phosphatase	21–93 u/L
Serum T4	58–128 u/L
Random blood sugar	3.4–9.3 mmol/L
SGOT	11–33 IU/L
LDH	58–145 IU/L
Bilirubin (men)	2–17 μmol/L
Bilirubin (women)	3–12 μmol/L
Urate (men)	0.19–0.31 mmol/L
Urate (women) +	0.13–0.46 mmol/L

Hospital admission

Because old people often feel that hospital admission is a 'one way ticket', it is necessary to explain carefully what it is hoped will be achieved and why you cannot manage the patient at home. This will, in many cases, be a mixture of clinical and social reasons. There is still a residual fear in some areas of the 'geriatric hospital'. It is often a good policy to arrange for a domiciliary visit from the consultant. This has the benefit of introducing the patient to the 'new doctor' and also of enabling the consultant to see the home to which he aims to return the patient.

What should be the content of the doctor's letter?

This is of particular importance in the elderly, who, not infrequently, find it difficult to give a good history, or even become confused by sudden transfer to the hospital environment. Also, in many cases, they are transported to hospital alone or with a person who knows little of their medical history.

The letter, therefore, should provide the fullest possible information in a concise manner. This is impossible for one who does not know the patient well, say a locum or deputizer.

Information should follow a certain form, and some practitioners have printed forms so that nothing is omitted.

Essential information to provide is:

(1) The reason for admission
Physical findings.
Provisional diagnosis.
(2) Relevant medical history.
Associated conditions, e.g. diabetes.
Surgical interventions and scars.
Relevant family history.
All medication, both prescribed and self-administered.
(3) Marital status, principal helper, next of kin.
Occupational status, all past occupations.
Mode of life, activity, interests.
Housing and neighbourhood.
Services provided
Note: 79% of patients in geriatric wards are aged 75 and over. 28% aged 85 and over.

The optimal discharge rate occurs in those areas with 7.6 to 10.5 beds per 1000 persons aged 65 and over.

Alternatives to admission

If no diagnosis is possible and there are no reasons for admitting the patient to hospital, the following routine is suggested:

- Visit frequently, in order to judge whether there is improvement, stability or deterioration, or further physical signs, e.g. malaena.
- Where investigation is difficult, e.g. in a patient who is anaemic for reasons unknown, a 24 h admission policy is very useful.
- If you have done a full assessment properly, then a domiciliary visit is unlikely to add more. Better to speak to your consultant on the telephone and he/she will then admit for planned investigation.
- Inspire confidence in relatives, i.e. that 'something is being done'.
- Work out a plan of care with the primary care team, e.g. daily collection of specimens, domiciliary physiotherapy, and engage family members in a caring role.

Be a personal doctor

The home of many an old person is a love object, so take the opportunity to meet them in it. Only then can you know them as a complete person. You may also note such things as cooking and bathing facilities, empty bottles of alcohol in odd corners, and home safety matters which can later be considered with the health visitor and nurse.

Even if they seem odd and eccentric, try to understand and respect old people. Do not push services on them before you have discussed whether they think they would be advantageous.

Always look after carers as well as the patients, since the majority of carers are registered with the same practice. The relationship between patient and carer is one of the symbiosis. Some comments made by carers to a research student are worth hearing, for they speak volumes:

> 'No, I haven't had any information, he's never suggested anything. If I ask, he is perfectly amenable but it would be nice for him to suggest things ....it would make you feel a bit more comfortable.'

> 'She has been very good when she has come. She listens, she doesn't rush off.'

> 'I don't like asking. I would prefer the doctor to volunteer information.'

'The fact he visits, psychologically does her good. Gives me moral support by talking to me.'

'Well, he hasn't really given us any information as such.'

HEALTH EDUCATION AND FOLLOW-UP

The elderly have been a generation unlike others in not having received health education. The wise doctor attempts to promote autonomy among his patients. Health education at each stage of follow-up is therefore important, nor need follow-up be carried out by the doctor. It will be required during the course of a chest infection, when examination of the lung bases, the sputum and PEF measurements need to be made, but once instruction has been given in rising slowly from recumbency to those suffering from postural hypotension, follow-up can be delegated to the nurse. Much has been achieved by the formation of stroke clubs, and even more may be achieved by a course of talks given to patients and their carers by team members at the practice premises.

Regular visiting of those at risk and the very old is desirable, but not always practical in districts heavily loaded with old people or in country practices spread over wide areas.

REFERENCES

Abraham, J. (1987). *Information Needs of Carers of Elderly People*. Community Health Council, Croydon

Hale, WE, Stewart, RB and Marks, RG. (1983). Haematological and biochemical laboratory values in an ambulatory elderly population: an analysis of the effects of age, sex and drugs. *Age Ageing*, 12, 275–284

Hodkinson, M. (1983). Biochemical changes in old age. *Med Int*, 1, (36), 1701–1703

Thompson, MK. (1972). *Update*, pp. 1005–1012

Thompson, MK. (1972). *Update*, pp. 1505–1513

Section 2
The Ageing Process

THE AGEING PROCESS

The epidemiology of ageing

In 1900, life expectancy at birth was 49 years; in 1949, about 68 years – a net gain of 19 years. But from 1950 to 1974, the gain has been only 3.8 years, and has continued to level off. We may wonder why there has been so great an increase in life expectancy in the first half of this century, but an equally profound levelling off in the beginning of the second half. We may be even more puzzled when considering that the extent of advances in biomedical research has been greater in the past 30 years than those made in all previous years. This apparent dilemma derives from the important distinction to be made between life expectancy and life span. The human life span, of about 100 years, has not changed since recorded history, but what has changed is the number of those surviving to the apparent limit, so that, in many privileged countries, you can now reasonably expect to become old, which is a very new phenomenon indeed. The challenge to mankind presented by this increase in life expectancy must be considered from the triple viewpoints of science, medicine and sociology as new obligations devolve on society to improve the quality of life for older people. It may be debated how much of this change has resulted from medical achievement and how much from improved social conditions, but, if the two leading current causes of death were resolved, the elimination of all vascular diseases and cancer would yield a net increase of about 19 years in life expectancy at birth, and only slightly less at age 65, a figure almost identical to the net increase in life expectancy achieved at birth in this country from 1900 to 1950. The increase in life expectancy at birth during the first half of this century resulted from the resolution of deaths which occurred before the age of 65, but the gain in life expectancy at ages 65 and 75 from 1900 to 1950 was, respectively, only 1.9 and 1.3 years, and from 1950–1974, 1.8 and 1.4 years. In a world in which all causes of death resulting from disease and accidents were totally eliminated, the effect on human longevity would be to realise the ultimate rectangular curve in which citizens would live without fear of premature death, but with the certain fate that on the eve of their one-hundreth birthday, they would die.

This situation is continuing to evolve because biomedical research has concentrated exclusively on the disease-associated causes of death. Scant attention has been paid to those underlying causes of biological ageing which are not disease associated but which, in clock-like fashion, dictate for each individual a specific maximum life span. Attention to such factors, logged from before birth and continuously as computerized data, would enable practitioners to use diagnosis effectively for prognosis, enabling advice on health promotion to be demonstrated.

The one comparatively innocuous way in which life expectancy can be significantly extended is by a calory-restricted diet. This has been demonstrated in animals and has been known for 50 years. It is of interest to note that no human has consciously chosen to follow this path, which is remarkable considering the many nostrums of other types that have been foisted on a gullible public. It suggests of course that, for most people, the quality of life is more important than its length.

Genetic aspects of ageing

The principal evidence that ageing is largely genetically determined is based upon the following observations:

1. *Life spans of specific species*
   Differences in life span of various animal groupings are strongly in favour of a species-specific genetic basis for longevity. Everyone knows about long-lived members of the turtle family, while, in mammals, the longest lived species is man (120 years) and the shortest lived species are small rodents: the golden hamster, for example, lives between 2 and 3 years.
2. *Hybrid vigour*
   Perhaps the best examples of the effect of genetic constitution on processes of ageing are accidentally incurred as a passive by-product of the genetic selection of advantageous properties, or indeed, that there are 'ageing genes' selected through evolution because they confer a direct advantage to survival of the species at the expense of the individual by an active process in slowing down, or shutting down vital processes.

We may conclude this section by considering two important biological principles. First, death from old age is almost certainly confined to man and domestic animals, for those in the wild are struck down by random causes – predators and accidental causes, well before they demonstrate the physiological decrements seen in very old humans. Man's success in dealing with his environment has therefore revealed a Pandora's box of vicissitudes never intended to be witnessed by him.

Ageing at cellular level

In 1961, Hayflick and Moorhead published their observations showing that human cell cultures had a limited replication life span. (The 'Hayflick Limit'). Later, the idea that this might serve as a model for the study of cellular ageing was supported by observations of a relationship between the age of the donor and culture longevity. But, in the case of the tissue most intensively studied, the human dermis, the extent of the regression is low, and the variance extremely high. Also, the pathobiology of ageing skin is probably a much less crucial determinant of lifespan in man than that of other tissues. Greater difficulty has been experienced in studies of other tissues, but there is now sufficient evidence from *in vitro* studies to suggest that all cell types seem to be involved in this decline.

Apart from the retardation of cell division with age, it has also been shown that there is a decrease, as a function of age, in the numbers of smooth muscle and endothelial cells capable of undergoing DNA synthesis, and it has been suggested that the myointimal proliferative lesions of atherosclerosis may result from a release of such cells from local regulatory inhibitory influences. Other apparently paradoxical proliferations are widespread within the ageing human, involving cartilage and synovial cells in osteoarthritis, prostatic epithelial and fibromuscular cells in benign prostatic hypertrophy, gliosis in the CNS, parenchymal fibrosis in the thyroid, regional obesity due to adipocytes, senile lentigos from melanocytes, and senile warts in epidermal cells.

Much of the diminution in psychosocial capability, which accompanies senescence, is interpreted as resulting from progressive impoverishment of the complicated interlacement of dendrites and axonal terminals surrounding the nerve cell bodies of the grey matter. The resulting loss of enormous numbers of synaptic connections results in progressive reduction in the computational power of the cerebral cortex and its programme library. The giant pyramidal cells of Betz appear particularly sensitive to the ageing process, for it can be shown that 60–75% of the total complement of Betz cells are damaged or destroyed by the 7th decade of life. The vast majority of Betz cells are located in portions of the motor cortex innervating the large extensor muscles of leg, thigh and trunk, with very little representation in the geographically more extensive zones concerned in hand, fingers, face and mouth. It has been suggested that the increasing stiffness of the lower extremities and the slowing of motor activity with age may be due in part to this progressive failure of Betz-cell activity.

Motor cells in the anterior horn of the spinal cord may show considerable change during the process of ageing, particularly the small motor neurones, the function of which is to maintain spindle patterns during periods when the surrounding muscle belly is unloaded. The combined result of such cell loss might well delay initiation of muscle contraction, and decrease the strength and precision of motor response, changes which characterize motor activity in the ageing individual. Secondary atrophic changes in muscle fibres, originally supplied by the dying neurons, result in decrease of total muscle mass and limitation of muscle strength and endurance, all commonly observed stigmata of the aged individual.

The biology of ageing and the ageing of physiological function

A lot of nonsense is talked about ageing. Insurance companies put the question to examining doctors 'Does the appearance of the candidate conform to the age given?' Presumably, conditions such as grey hair, wrinkles and body posture are sought, but even if present they are an uncertain guide. The practitioner, nevertheless, regards age as important data in patient management, and will note the considerable difference between chronological and biological age which will be relative, rather than related to a standard, and measured more in terms of performance than by clinical testing.

In paediatrics, we are able to measure milestones of development. These are so regular that concern is caused if they are not reached within a short period of time. In the late decades, the biological differences between individuals is diverse enough to make many fail to realise that development still continues, but very slowly. We may think then of the child as 'ageing' very rapidly, and the old person, very slowly. It would be better to abandon the term 'ageing' with its emotional overtones, and to use the term 'development' instead.

The progress of senescence is often described as 'degeneration' but it is necessary to see the manifestations so described as a result of changes in homeostasis without which development cannot take place. In old age, such changes produce frailty as the internal environment is by then so distorted that vulnerability is greatly increased. The practice of medicine has moved away from the 19th century model, when an ecological model prevailed, and diseases were produced in vast numbers by micro-organisms and dietary deficiencies. Such diseases, the result of a hostile environment, were defined and classified, and medical skills depended on accurate diagnosis and finesse in distinguishing one from another. Increasingly now we are concerned with a relatively few conditions which can be measured against norms in assessing health prospects, such as blood pressure and blood cholesterol. The extension of the life span of the average person has taken place during the phase of immaturity rather than at the end. Many phenomena are better managed by monitoring and gentle control, rather than by heroic intervention. Increasingly, attention is paid to the management of the lifestyle of the patient.

We may also seek to understand the different patterns of disease in the elderly. These are:

>Multiple pathology,
>Insidious onset of disease,
>Atypical presentation
>Unexpected recovery.

In a study of more than 600 patients in general practice on whom there were complete records, eight conditions emerged with such regularity that they appeared to parallel the milestones of development in childhood because, if more than one was not present by the age of 70, it could be doubted whether the individual was ageing normally! I called these the eight diseases of ageing, though strictly they are not diseases but altered states of physiology which, if not controlled, lead to organ damage and complications. These diseases of ageing, while more common in the elderly, are not exclusive to them, and are in fact more serious in young people so far as prognosis is concerned. They were, in my own practice:

>Obesity,
>Atherosclerosis,
>Diabetes type II,
>Hypertension,
>Cancer,
>Endogenous depression,
>Auto-immune disease,
>Immunological failure.

One is immediately struck by several features of this list. First of all, they all have features in common, suggesting that there might be a common factor in the pathogenesis. Thus, one condition, such as obesity, may predispose to another condition, such as diabetes or hypertension.

Secondly, it follows that the management of one condition may be best achieved by control of another. Thus, the first thing one decides to do when meeting a hypertensive who is obese, is control the obesity and monitor the blood pressure.

Thirdly, all these diseases are of uncertain aetiology, although clinically more commonly found with advancing age. In each one, however, one can be sure that they evolve long before they cross the clinical threshold and produce symptoms.

Finally, I found 86% of those aged over 70 in my practice population had these diseases present, not singly, but almost always in combination (after accounting for 12% of accidental deaths). It now becomes important to acquire new clinical attitudes, looking for overlap instead of diagnosing single diseases by exclusion. So we must bear in mind that hypertension has higher incidence among diabetics than non-diabetics. Hyperinsulinaemia promotes cell division, obesity is linked metabolically with cancer, atherosclerosis and diabetes. This theme could be greatly developed. But it becomes clear why the management of one condition by control of another assumes major importance in the old, while controlling unfavourable life-styles becomes the basis of prevention in those of younger age.

This theme could be greatly expanded, but what it does suggest is that there is a regulator of development, or a biological clock.

Human development and gerontology

The general principle behind the maintenance of a stable internal environment is negative feedback control, which works throughout a number of systems, common to which is the hypothalamus (Figure 2.1). Thus, what is generally regarded as the entry to adult life, the activation of the reproductive system, occurs more in relation to weight than to age. From studies in anorexia nervosa, it has been pointed out that menstruation occurs when a critical weight of 48 kg is reached. This can be affected by interference with food intake, the appetite and satiety centre being intimately linked in the hypothalamus with LRH. Female development provides further information with the event in middle life, the menopause, which has occurred at a regular age of 50–51 since medieval times. Such striking constancy of factors associated with human development, and the regular finding of older people suffering from eight overlapping diseases, suggest that ageing is governed by regular patterns and hormonal shifts, rather than by probability factors.

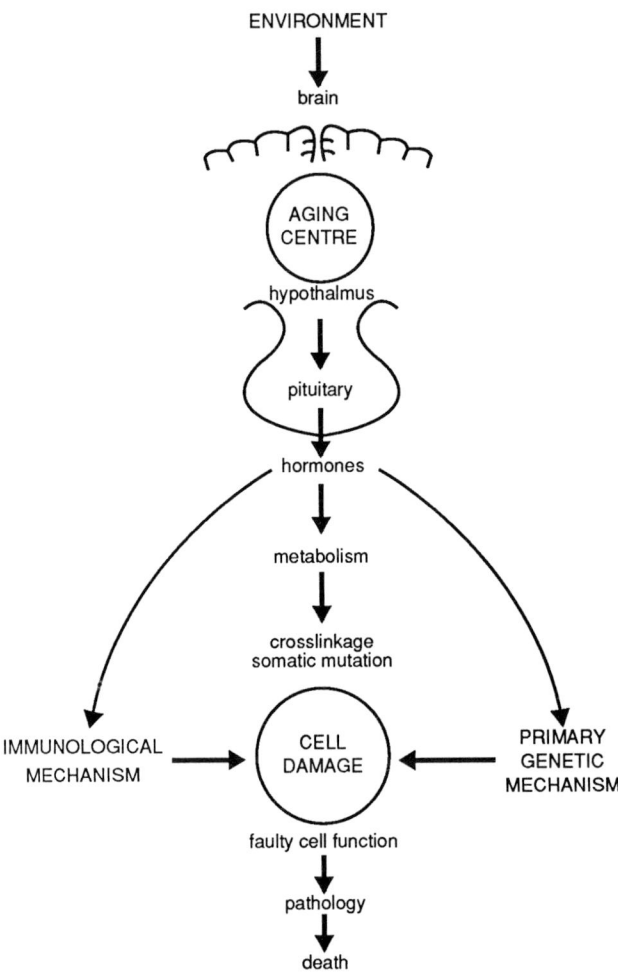

Figure 2.1 The role of the pituitary in regulating aging processes. The rate of aging (or cell damage) is primarily under genetic control, but is modified by environmental factors acting via neuroendocrine mechanisms. It is postulated that information from the environment (both internal and external) is relayed to an aging centre in the hypothalamus which regulates the rate of aging by altering the secretion of pituitary and other hormones. The hormones interact with metabolic, immunological, and genetic mechanisms of aging.

The energy and reproductive homeostats

These are linked together in this section simply because, in the dynamic state of daily living, they interact.

The energy homeostat is concerned with carbohydrates and animal fats as fuel or energy producing substrates. The energy homeostat can be seen as a four-component model with two main hormones controlling the utilization of these substrates, insulin and glucose, and growth hormone (GH) controlling the utilization of free fatty acids (FFA). In many ways, these two mechanisms are antagonistic. During the day, it is mainly glucose which is used for energy supply, and it is not necessary to draw upon energy reserves stored in fat depots as triglycerides. At the same time, glucose stimulates the secretion of insulin, which exerts an antilipolytic effect on the one hand, and ensures the utilization of glucose on the other. Conversely, at night, when no food is eaten, the energy supply is switched over to the predominant use of FFA instead of glucose, the level of which falls in the blood, thus leading to a rise in GH level and a decline in blood insulin level. The increase in blood level of FFA, which is chiefly taken up by muscle tissue for energy supply also suppresses glucose uptake for this purpose, thus contributing to a better supply of glucose to nervous tissues (Figure 2.2).

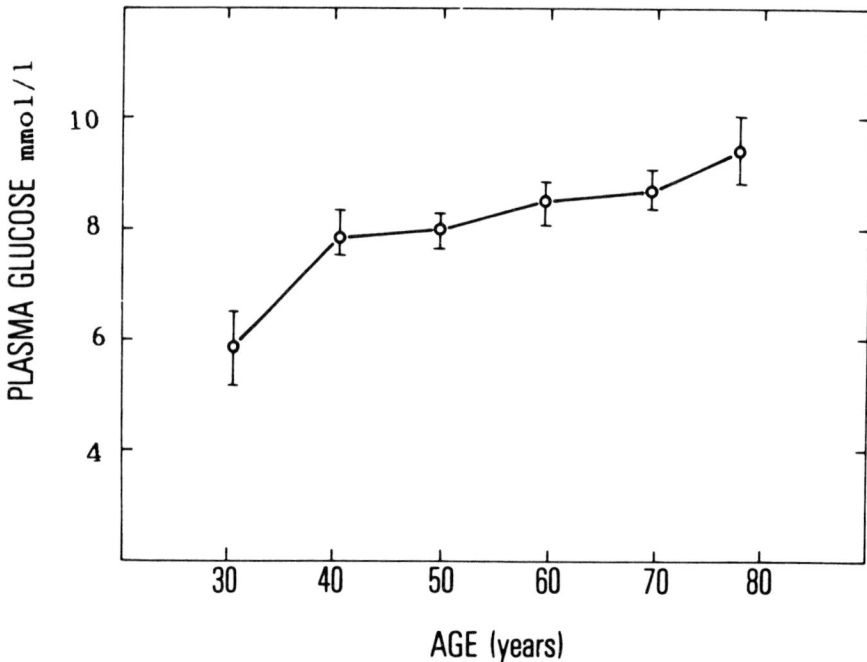

Figure 2.2 Effect of age on plasma glucose concentration 2 hours after oral glucose. Clean group. For each decade from 30–80 were 14, 50, 82, 67, 53, and 33.

There are, of course, eventually many other regulatory effects on energy processes: for instance, glucocorticoids have effects similar to that of growth hormone, reducing glucose uptake by muscle tissue. It is necessary to understand the rudiments of these processes in order to understand metabolic changes inherent in ageing as fat accumulates and lean body mass is reduced. These age-dependent dynamics include: glucose intolerance; increased blood cholesterol, triglyceride, beta-lipoprotein and insulin levels; and an increase in reactive hyperinsulinaemia which develops after glucose loading. It is generally explained that such age-related metabolic changes are caused by external factors such as excessive food intake, low physical activity and stress, and, although it is true that these play an important role, it is not only these external factors which determine changes in energy regulation. This explains why it is so difficult to control excess weight, particularly in older females in whom there is a disturbed rhythm in the function of the energy homeostat, resulting in the central type of homeostatic failure. It is notable, for instance, that young people react to stress by loss of appetite, whereas older people tend to eat excessively. The domination of the glucose or diurnal type of regulation is gradually superseded by the domination of the fat or nocturnal type of regulation. As age advances with a rise in the hypothalamic threshold of sensitivity to glucose, postprandial glycaemia produces compensatory insulinaemia which does not arrest the decline in glucose utilization completely. Therefore, tolerance to carbohydrates gradually diminishes, and hyperinsulinaemia, in conjunction with an excessive glucose level, stimulates triglyceride synthesis, leading to the development of age-associated obesity. This produces metabolic shifts and a second cycle of disturbance because free fatty acid utilization inhibits glucose uptake by muscle tissue. This closed cycle can be regarded as the 'fat shunt'. In summary, glucose taken with food is not fully used by muscle tissue and hyperinsulinaemia converts further carbohydrate sources into fat. The deposits are drawn upon, and fatty acids, often in excess, are channeled to the target tissues, and metabolic conditions similar to those in maturity-onset diabetes are created. Carried to this stage, the metabolic disturbances can no longer return to normal. While fats burn in the flames of carbohydrates, the reverse is not the case, and a vicious circle of age-associated disturbances is formed.

The predominant utilization of fatty acids as a source of energy is inherent not only in normal ageing, but in such age-specific disorders as atherosclerosis, metabolic immunodepression, diabetes type II, obesity and cancer. Thus, the human organism, in the final analysis, burns in the flame of fats.

The female menopause, unique to the human species, is the most clear cut example of endocrine senescence, terminating reproductive function at an age beyond which childbearing would be hazardous. Blood levels and urinary excretion of oestrogen decline after the age of forty, and continue to decline further between ages 50 and 60, reaching a level in the elderly about one fifth of that before the menopause. In obese women, the menopause may be delayed due to enhancement of conversion of increased amounts of adrenal androstenedione to oestrogen in the periphery in partial compensation for ovarian failure.

It is difficult to support the hypothesis that ovarian failure and the origin of the menopause lies in the ovaries when considerable follicular reserve still remains. The failure to suppress gonadotropins to premenopausal levels, despite hormone replacement therapy to restore premenopausal levels, supports the concept of central failure in the reproductive homeostat. At puberty, the decrease in sensitivity of the sex centre to inhibition by sex hormones constitutes a fundamental change leading to enhanced activity of the hypothalamus, gonadal development, sexual maturity and reproductive function. It seems reasonable to apply Occam's razor, and to consider that the same mechanism of hypothalamic insensitivity produces the menopause. The fact that, years before the menopause, there is an essential change in the LH to FSH ratio, in favour of the latter which eventually becomes excessive, suggests that a high level of FSH (by which the menopause is diagnosed in problematic cases) harmfully affects the follicular tissue of the ovaries, while a raised level of LH, by causing thecal hyperplasia, changes the spectrum of the hormones produced. The relief of hot flushes and other menopausal discomforts by HRT is not due to the replaced hormones themselves, but to the reduction in autonomic effects from hypothalamic activity partially controlled by negative feedback.

Age-associated changes in the male reproductive system are characterized by certain distinctive features. Firstly, the cyclic centre does not function in the male organism. Secondly, although the reproductive function is switched on by a mechanism in the hypothalamus, no mechanism is provided for switching it off. The age-associated decrease in the reproductive ability of males is caused by the lowered level of sex hormones, leading to diminished potency. Blood testosterone level starts to decrease after the age of 50, although a high level of testosterone, typical of young men, may be observed in men 80 or even 90 years old. Phenomena similar to the climacteric do not occur.

In the female organism, the oestrogen level is raised in obesity, inhibiting the development of age-associated atherosclerosis which is one example of many differences in ageing between the two sexes.

Of the intrinsic theories of ageing, there are two categories. Firstly, random causes, such as somatic mutation, error catastrophe, free-radical theory, cross-linkage theory, immunological theory, and others. But ageing is characterized by a striking constancy of manifestations, so that all of these theories have limitations. The regular development of such metabolic shifts as age-associated fat accumulation, hyperinsulinaemia and hypercholesterolaemia, and such hormonal shifts as the climacteric promote the idea of a specific pattern of ageing and age pathology. For instance, while immunological theory provides some explanation of the development of such processes as cancer and age-associated autoimmune phenomena, it fails to account for the formation of such functional processes as the climacteric or mental depression.

Of the control theories, cell theories, such as the 'Hayflick Limit' which set certain limits to the number of possible cell divisions in each species of animal, fail to account for changes occurring in the regulatory system, since neurons do not divide in the adult organism. There is much to favour a more universal concept of the regularities of human ageing and development and diseases of ageing. Whereas embryonic development, cellular differentiations and growth entail programmed, non-damaging interaction, age-dependent disorders appear to result from errors that occur in central control systems which subsequently give rise to strong pathogenic interactions. Ageing is conceived as linked with the inevitability of changes, and, of course, in the elderly, diseases exist as a continuum of severity, and not as an 'all-or-none' phenomenon.

It is worth noting, in conclusion, that the efficiency of cell-mediated immunity decreases with advancing age. In contrast, the capacity for autoantibody synthesis does not appear to be depressed with ageing. Thus, on the one hand, there is a reduction in numbers, or at least cellular immune response, of T-cells, while older humans exhibit a rise in the incidence of autoantibodies.

With regard to the ' diseases of ageing', therefore, it is worth pointing out that they are not the cause, but, to a considerable degree, the sequelae of the increasing vulnerability of the ageing organism. Thus, over the past 200 years, the life expectancy of humans once the age of 60 has been reached, has altered a little. On a population basis, therefore, western societies are, in a sense, reaching the limits of medical progress unless the process of ageing itself can be influenced. For this reason, geriatric medicine is concerned with maladies that have an age-specific peak incidence in relation to the downswing of the survival curve.

Changes in appearance and function

We are accustomed daily to observing changes such as wrinkling of the skin, greying of the hair and frontal balding. They are so common that, by the age of 50, half the population has greying hair. Body fat is redistributed centrally, with peripheral changes, such as guttering of the interossei, and the appearance suggesting enophthalmos, due to loss of fat in the orbit.

The eyes

By the age of 48, most normally-sighted people will need 1 dioptre reading glasses, increasing up to about 3 dioptres in the early 60's. This is due to one of the linear age changes in which the lens begins to harden from the age of 6 onwards, presbyopic changes being noticed in the forties when the normal reading distance of 25 cm is lengthened, particularly in poor light. Other changes that occur are a loss of colour discrimination, particularly between green and blue, and a slowing of adaptation to darkness.

Hearing

There is a loss of high-frequency sounds, such as consonants like 's' and 't' which makes the spoken word particularly difficult to comprehend when there is background noise. Speech sounds are distorted, rather than lacking in volume, which is why raising the voice may be met with the admonishment: 'There is no need to shout, young man. I am not deaf!'

The understanding of speech is, of course, a cerebral activity. Compensation for what is not heard clearly is gained by observation of facial expression and hand gesture. Speaking to an older person requires two considerations by the speaker: first, that speech should not be rapid, and words should be clear and simple. Secondly, one should sit in a quiet room, on the same level, and wait until an alert posture has been adopted on the part of the listener, making sure that one's own face is in the light and clearly visible. Then, speech should be made at a reasonable pace, using short sentences with a gap between, accentuating syllables and making full use of gesture and expression. Such an achievement may be rewarded by the grateful retort: 'You are the only person I can understand properly'. Hearing aids have a use in amplifying sound. In presbyacusis, this can make things worse.

Changes in function

Of the decline of functional capacity that for physical work is the function most reduced by age. Between the ages of 30 and 75, the capacity for sustained heavy work is reduced by 60%, but the maximal effort is reduced by only 30%. However, on average, changes over time in the performance of different organ systems proceed at different rates, indicating clearly that each subject must be evaluated on a variety of performances. In general, however, the percentage decrement in some functions, such as nerve conduction velocity, is less than others, such as vital capacity, and still less than maximal work rate and oxygen uptake, the last being reduced by 70% compared with the performance of the average 30-year-old.

In order to validate an index of functional age, it will be necessary to collect repeated observations on subjects throughout the life cycle, a function reserved, perhaps, for general practice. We may be able to identify subjects who are 'young for their age' but we cannot know whether the apparent delay in age changes in middle or early old age, is a reflection of a slower rate of ageing in the individual. There are many tests for which a score can be devised to characterise the deviation of the performance of an individual from the mean value of a group of his age peers. Tests which have been used in a number of studies include:

> Systolic blood pressure,
> Diastolic blood pressure,
> Hearing loss,
> Vital capacity,
> Reaction time,
> Grip strength,
> Visual acuity,
> Accomodation of the eye,
> FEV,
> Vibratory sensitivity,

Metacarpal osteoporosis index (females),
Skin elasticity,
Side flexion,
Picture recognition,
Tapping rate.

However, different workers have found a wide range of correlation coefficients with age among the different studies, reflecting perhaps sample differences in the populations tested.

Psychological aspects of ageing

There is a psychology of every age, so that comparing the mental performance of the young with the old is like comparing chalk and cheese. It is perhaps impossible to isolate mental performance from the motivating forces within a social setting. The best example of mental change with age is memory, but so common is the forgetting of names by the age of 40 (the benign senescent forgetfulness of Kral), that is a matter for social amusement rather than individual concern. In general, memory loss should be regarded as a symptom of disease rather than a feature of ageing.

If we consider mental function throughout human development, we note that language learning by children up to the age of three involves a faculty largely forfeited by the age of 20. It is also clear that teenage years are largely spent in the search for personal identity and testing parental influence against that of peer judgement. Educational systems are designed to enable the young to learn in order to establish themselves in society. When Frances Carp tested the theory that behavioural characteristics commonly perceived as 'senile traits' are indicators of adjustment, and not specific to the late years of life, she compared a group of college students with a group of elderly people, and found the students showed more neurosis, negativism, dissatisfaction, and a higher proportion of socially inept persons with unrealistic and unfavourable views of themselves. The appearance of such symptoms as unusual nervousness, irritability, depression, unaccountable anger, personality change, apathy of withdrawal, the taking of drugs and wearing dirty uncared-for clothing, are considered in the young to be clear indications for psychotherapy; in the elderly, they are frequently considered par for the course of old age. They are, of course, indicators of adjustment by the young and the old who are alternately courting the favours of a rejecting society, and expressing hostility to it. Studies in social deprivation have shown, even in the young, the need for continual confrontation with reality, and particularly for the kind of social interaction where conversation allows verbalization of sensory input to make differentiation possible between intrinsic and extrinsic stimuli. Lone sailors, pot holers and widows alike hallucinate because of the projection of inner feelings into a fantasy reality.

It is important to recognize, and to make allowance for, social variants. It is doubtful if isolation is always harmful in a rapidly changing society, or a marked sign of personality deviation. There have always existed life-long isolates for whom being alone represents a way of life, and hardy and adaptable people exist for whom solitude is a necessary condition for stability. They may find the problems that they have to face preferable to the perpetuated shallowness of attending the bingo hall.

The age decrement in mental ability probably arises as an interaction between an intrinsic adverse biological process and the cumulative effect of injury and disease. The result is a decline in a wide range of cognitive functions which is particularly evident in tasks where a solution

> Our attention in the practice was directed towards a 74-year-old widower who had moved into a block of council flats but appeared to be on no doctor's list. The reason for being asked to see him was that he appeared mentally disturbed and was constantly made fun of by groups of children who gathered to jeer at him as he returned from the shops. The cause of their merriment was that he doffed his hat with great politeness and greeted a bush standing outside the entrance. Examination showed that he had bilateral cataract so advanced that he could not distinguish the bush from the human figure which had become familiar to him. In one way, it was fortunate that inspissated wax and sensorineural deafness had made him very deaf, so that he did not hear the mockery, but it had completed his isolation from sensory stimuli. After cleaning his ears, supplying a hearing aid, and having the cataracts extracted, he was able to laugh at his misfortune, and join a working man's club where he was respected as a fine darts player. He was poorly nourished, and temporarily impaired by sensory deprivation, but recovered well.

to a problem has to be provided within a given time. Some of this retardation of response is due to delay within the central nervous system, but it must be realized that, whereas young people love to shine, the elderly fear to fail, particularly having reached an age when speed has become unnecessary. This may also account for another characteristic of old people, which is mental rigidity, and a relative inability to look at situations in new ways, which, when applied to personal relationships can make such people difficult to live with, and may be a barrier to successful rehabilitation when new ways of living have to be learned.

Impairment of short-term memory is a well-known failure in the elderly, so the same object may be repeatedly lost. It seems as though the mind has evolved a technique for conserving important memory without becoming saturated with trivia, but that the faculty for holding information, such as a shopping list, for a short time only may become impaired once one has come to reply upon routine living. On the other hand, the loss of this faculty may simply be due to cellular changes in the cerebrum.

Old people learn to react to intellectual decline by avoiding those tasks which impose an intolerable strain on their brain power, and, if confronted by an overtaxing situation, they will replace appropriate cerebral activity by inappropriate motor responses, such as scratching the head or losing their temper. This response can take dramatic form with widespread autonomic manifestations, verbal tirade, tears or total silence. Doctors should learn to recognize this catastrophic reaction and avoid provoking it.

There is evidence that certain kinds of verbal learning are well retained and more resistant to the normal effects of ageing than other mental skills. The retention of adequate vocabulary may therefore allow substantial losses of mental ability to pass undetected without special testing. Thus there are those in old age, even in their 80's and 90's, who preserve their intellectual powers and personality intact. At the other end of the spectrum are the legions of the depressed and demented whose life is contracted, weakened and fragmented. It is possible to suggest indices by which this latter group at special risk of mental breakdown might be identified:

> Advanced age,
> Poor physical health,
> Impairment of the special senses,
> Reduced mobility and capacity for self care,

Moodiness, anxiety or hypochondriasis in the premorbid personality,
History of previous mental illness in patient or relatives,
Low sociability,
For every day contacts/decreasing frequency of social visiting,
Limited range of interests in the past.

Effects of environmental factors and life patterns on life span

The consensus of scientific opinion is that the fundamental underlying causes of age changes, like developmental changes, are somehow programmed within the genetic apparatus, but that their expression can be influenced by extrinsic factors. Health education is based upon principles which, if not observed, hasten the appearance of diseases which are basically intrinsic in origin, and the strategy for preventing or retarding the onset of these diseases is that of retarding or modifying biological ageing. The four pillars on which health education is based is the avoidance of over-eating, under-exercising, smoking and stress.

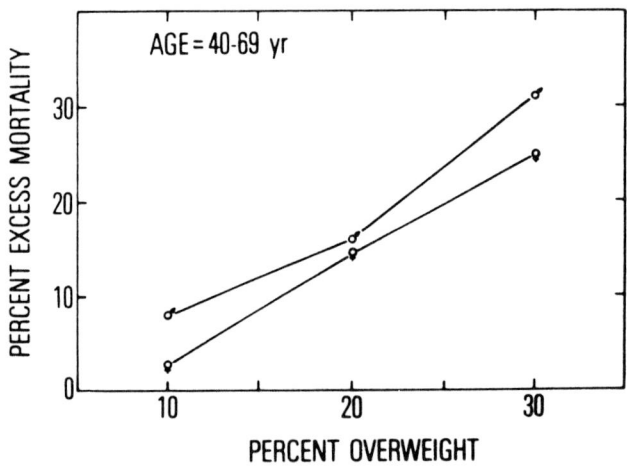

Figure 2.3 Effect of overweight on excess mortality. The data are from the Society of Actuaries Building and Blood Pressure Study 1959. The figure is drawn from data for 'Cases without known minor impairments' and includes subjects who 'were insured either as standard risks, or were rated as substandard risks only because of weight, having no other impairment that would bar them from obtaining standard insurance' (*Stat. Bull.*, Feb., 1960, p.8, and Mar., 1960, p.2).

The influence of obesity

Obesity has been shown to be associated with major life-shortening illnesses, such as coronary heart disease, hypertension and diabetes (Figure 2.3), while Wynder (1976) has shown experimentally that a fat-rich diet may intensify carcinogenesis. Excess glucose, unutilized by muscle tissue, is taken up by the adipose tissue for triglyceride synthesis. Consequently body weight, or to be more precise, body fat content, increases with ageing. The resultant increased utilization of free fatty acids as energy substrates leads also to increased risk of thrombogenesis, but in particular metabolic immunodepression. Food intake is normally regulated chiefly through the mediation of glucose which binds to the glucoreceptors of the hypothalamic satiety centre. For this reason, it is interesting to note that, in general, when the young are stressed, appetite is inhibited; in the elderly, the reverse often occurs, with consequent consumption of food, such as biscuits.

Large insurance studies by the Society of Actuaries have emphasized the continuous direct relationship between obesity and mortality extending over the entire distribution of relative body weight except, perhaps, for those extremely underweight. However, the 'ideal' or 'desirable' body weight for middle-aged and elderly adults is considerably higher than that presented in the most commonly used height–weight tables. In fact, the techniques available for quantification of obesity for ordinary purposes rely upon the obesity index and skinfold thickness since there are no criteria for classifying an individual's frame size.

Using such criteria, the Framington Study noted that minimal mortality occurred in the men at an obesity index level of 1.25 to 1.39, whereas a longitudinal study of 14 years by the Chicago Gas Company noted that the minimal mortality for the 50–59 year age group occurred at an obesity index of 1.25 to 1.32 (Figure 2.4). Other studies have produced either similar results or no striking effect of obesity on mortality.

We might conclude from this that physicians should reconsider urging the general public that minor deviations in weight from the sacrosanct 'desirable weight' tables will doom one to an early grave. We are quite accustomed to hearing that in affluent societies obesity is the number one health problem. We know from experience that the therapy of obesity is dismal indeed. The impact of this health advice on the anxiety levels of many older people is difficult to measure, and the impact of

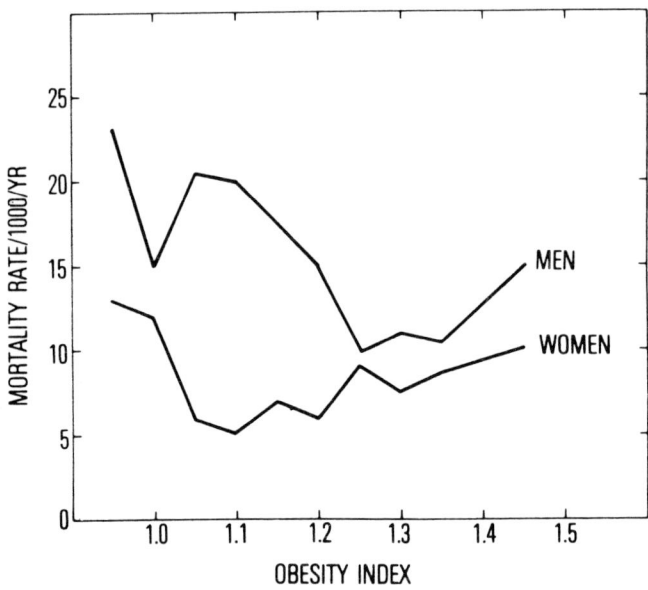

Figure 2.4 Relation of obesity to mortality – The Framingham Study. The mortality rate is reported as the annual incidence per 1000 population at risk at examination (Kannel and Gordon 1974). Data for men and women are grouped for ages 45–74 y. The data plotted at obesity index 1.0, 1.1 etc. represent the subjects who ranged from 1.00 to 1.04, 1.10 to 1.14

this anxiety on the development of other diseases and on the general sense of well-being is also unknown.

The literature is heavy with articles and book chapters on the risks and hazards of obesity. There must be another side to the coin. It behoves us to provide more realistic standards for judging obesity than those so readily available to the public and physicians. The screening procedure is as available as the nearest bathroom scale. We require of screening programmes of disease and risk factors that the perils of the factor be clearly demonstrated, that the screening technique be accurate, and that something can be done about the risk factor when it is correctly identified.

A gain in body weight occurs in normal subjects with advancing age. Some causes of this are age-connected hyperglycaemia and hyperinsulinaemia, diminished muscular activity, and excessive food intake, particularly of carbohydrates, as a result of the disturbed regulation of appetite, factors which tend to shift metabolism toward fat accumulation. With ageing, man does not start putting on more weight because he eats more, but he eats more because he stores fat. Weight increase in men is maximal from 40–49 years, but in women a decade later.

The role of exercise in ageing

The largest deterioration in physical work capacity related to age takes place in cardiovascular and respiratory function. There have been a number of reports of the decrement in maximal oxygen intake with age as an objective measure of cardiorespiratory performance. But there is less evidence available describing the rate of decrease of aerobic capacity, or the ability to deliver oxygen to working muscle as affected by regular participation in exercise. However, longitudinal studies have indicated that sedentary men had a significantly greater annual decrement in the VO_2 max than habitually active individuals. The circulatory effects of endurance conditioning on sedentary middle aged and older men have been examined. After a training programme of three one half-hour periods of running per week for 8 to 10 weeks, VO_2max increased an average of 14%, maximal cardiac output increased by 13% and heart rate was lower during submaximal exercise, stroke volume increased by 16% at maximal exercise, and mean arterial blood pressure was on the average 5 mmHg lower. These men were aged 38 to 55. Exercise conditioning of older men aged 52–88 showed a significant increase in the integrated work output up to heart rate of 90% of maximum, significant reduction in resting systolic and diastolic blood pressure, and significant increases in strength of elbow flexion, vital capacity, and minute volume. From this it might be concluded that the trainability of older men with respect to physical work capacity and fitness is probably greater than had been suspected. Reviews of Soviet literature on physical activity and ageing indicate that improvement was most marked at the end of 3 to 5 years in respect of strength, balance and jumping in place.

Some interesting studies have been done on joint stiffness, by oscillation of the index finger passively about its metacarpophalangeal joint. These showed that there was significantly greater joint stiffness in old men than the young, but no significance between the two groups in measured strength. After a six-week training programme, significant increases in strength and decreases in joint stiffness were seen in both the young and older groups, and it was concluded that joint stiffness in both young and old men, in the absence of arthritis or other joint disease, is

> A woman of 78, living alone, admitted two men who told her they had to examine a tree in her garden which was dangerous. Once in the home, she was bound to a chair, gagged, and her money and possessions stolen. Some hours later, she was found by a friend, and a medical visit requested. She was not known to be hypertensive or diabetic, but an examination showed BP 190/120, and there was glycosuria, with a trace of proteinuria. Next morning, a random blood sugar was taken, showing a level of 14 mmol/L. It was decided not to label this lady 'diabetic' but to take daily sugar and blood pressure readings. After three weeks, the levels gradually fell back to normal for her.

a reversible phenomenon, suggesting the need to reconsider our ideas concerning the trainability of older individuals.

An extensive and interesting review by Montoye (1974) of the effects of exercise on longevity compared the age at death of men who participated in athletics during their youth with those who did not, revealing little difference in life expectancy for former college athletic award winners compared with their college class mates. He suggested, however, that regular engagement in physical activity, and control of body weight, throughout life may be more important in the mesomorphic (athletic) body type compared with others in order to maintain a healthy cardiovascular system.

The advice given to old people concerning exercise is superficial and extremely vague, varying between recommendations to 'take things easy' or 'be more active'. Old people do not find it easy to take exercise, particularly if they do not have a garden and live in towns. They will also have received different advice from different doctors, set against a cultural background which is very slowly changing away from inactive leisure pursuits. It is the doctor who will best judge an exercise programme for an individual, tailoring it to their requirements, ensuring that they will enjoy it and providing information on what facilities are available in the area. The physical and psychological benefits of physical fitness are great, but unfortunately, for a number of reasons, older people lag far behind what is attainable.

Smoking

In my own practice, I studied the smoking habits of 150 women in relation to the time of the menopause, repeating the work of Jick *et al.* (1977) who had found that, even making allowance for the normally later menopause of obese women, women who smoke have an earlier menopause than non-smokers. The findings were that the majority of women who smoked were postmenopausal before the age of 50, while non-smokers were grouped heavily between 50 and 51.

The RCGP oral contraception study showed an increased risk of arterial diseases in smokers compared with controls, mostly in older women.

Osteoporosis is more common in women who smoke than in non-smokers.

Tyler and his colleagues (1984) found, in general practice, that patients with malignant diseases of all kinds, other than skin cancer, smoked more than controls.

These findings suggest a wider effect than that smoking is a causative factor in bronchial carcinoma and ischaemic heart disease. Rather they suggest that smoking increases the rate of ageing, bringing forward in time the occurrence of diseases of ageing defined as deviations of homeostasis in the internal environment. We know that smoking raises the blood pressure, increases the heart rate, and daily smokers have higher serum cholesterol levels than non-smokers. It is important to remember, therefore, when considering that cancer incidence is directly proportional to the time of exposure, in patients who smoke exposure time flies faster because of the intensification of normal ageing processes.

As has been pointed out elsewhere, there have been relatively small gains in life expectancy at ages over 50 or 60 in the past 200 years. The real dangers of smoking are in early life, since it is there that the extension of longevity has taken place. So far as advising older people, the recommendation to abandon smoking has other reasons: chiefly physical fitness, social acceptance, and financial. Nevertheless, in general practice, the patient thinks of the present, and the doctor nearly always of the future. Advice to young people is of particular importance, since, barring accidents, they too will become old. The reduction of mortality ratio of coronary heart disease is relatively modest compared with that of lung cancer. The percentages have plateau'd in recent years for teenage boy and girl smokers, and it is this cohort of the future that risks impeding improvement in longevity.

Stress and accelerated ageing

No doctor is more involved with the effect of stress on patient health than the GP. Yet there is poor general understanding of its significance. Even a book on Prevention of Disease in the Elderly does not mention it. No one will have failed to recognize relationships between stress and diseases of ageing, such as hypertension, glycosuria, cancer, depression and so on. Nor will it have been unobserved that the young seem to seek deliberately after danger, exposure, conflict and other forms of stress, while the elderly seek to avoid it at all costs. I suggest that stress is a potent accelerator of the ageing process. In one group it is pursued in a race towards the advantages of adulthood; in the other, ageing slowly, it would be folly to accelerate decline.

Be that as it may, stress is difficult to define because we cannot easily judge it in others. We need to recognize that stress may be experienced through under promotion just as much as from promotion, so that one is only under stress if one feels under stress.

We know from the work of Selye and Tuchweber that, in the general adaptation syndrome, the organism fails to maintain the same level of resistance to stress throughout the lifespan. We may ask, why is the amount of adaptation energy finite, and subject to exhaustion under the influence of stress? Why is the intensity of the stress reaction, or, to be more precise, the time required for it to subside, increased during the course of ageing?

Two youths, beaten over the head in the town and robbed, were examined. In each case, blood pressure readings had risen to 150/95, and blood sugar readings were 10.6 and 9.4 respectively, although no food had been taken for three hours. The next day, blood pressures were 125/80 and 115/70, and blood sugars three hours after breakfast were 6.4 and 5.8 mmol/L.

The mechanism of reaction to stress is actuated by intensification of the hypothalamic–pituitary–adrenal complex. This involves disturbances of homeostasis, such as increased blood levels of cortisol, fatty free acids and glucose. Such increased levels in the blood of substances exerting negative feedback mechanisms inhibit the hypothalamic–pituitary complex, so that in cases of chronic stress, the defence mechanism against stressors undergoes a decrease in sensitivity and an elevation of the threshold at which receptor cells in the hypothalamus respond.

It is interesting, here, to consider the commonly observed relationship between chronic stress and depression, for it has been observed that some patients with endogenous depression oversecrete cortisol, and do not suppress its secretion when given dexamethasone. MAO levels increase in the brain with age, and numerous epidemiological studies have established that the prevalence of depression increases with age. The role of stress in malignancy has been considered to be the result of immunodepression related to biochemical changes, which, in turn, suppress cell-mediated immunity.

Changes causing a shift in the energy supply system are indispensable for defence against stress. We have all seen patients, who having nursed a spouse through terminal illness, succumb themselves within a few months, leaving us with the feeling that one event had led to the other. Stress, therefore, not only brings about mental depression, but also accelerates normal ageing, in one instance by a decrease in biogenic amine level, and the other by an elevation of the hypothalamic threshold of response to negative feedback. Middle-aged and older patients respond to surgical stress with longer rises in blood 11-hydroxycorticosteroid level than younger ones. One therefore pays a higher price for protection from stress in old age than in youth. But we shall never abolish stress from our own lives, or the lives of our patients. Death is inevitable, presumably because life is stressful, and one may conclude with the pessimistic note that we should die from its effects even in a perfect environment.

REFERENCES

Montoye, HJ. (1974). *Science and Medicine of Exercise and Sport*, 2nd Edn (New York: Harper and Row)

Andres, R. (1981). Influence of obesity on longevity in the aged. *Ageing: A Challenge to Science and Society, Vol.1 Biology. (Oxford University Press)*

Jick, *et al.* (1977). Relation between smoking and age of natural menopause. *Lancet*, 1, 1354

Tyler, SJ *et al.* (1984). Smoking and malignant disease: a general practice study. *J R Coll Gen Practit*, 34, 589–592

Johnson, WM. (1947). Different weight response to the same provocation. *J Am Med Assoc*, 133, 1238

Selye, H and Tuchweber, B. (1976). Stress in relation to ageing and disease. In Everitt, AV and Burgess, JA (eds) *Hypothalamus, Pituitary and Ageing*, pp.553–569. (Springfield, Ill: Charles C Thomas)

Wynder, EL. (1976). Nutrition and cancer. *Proc Soc Exp Biol Med*, 35, 1309–1315

Hayflick, L and Moorehead, PS. (1961). *Exp Cell Res*, 25, 585

Thompson, MK. (1986). The case for developmental gerontology – Thompson's Octad. *J R Coll Gen Practit*, 36, 29–32

Carp, FM. (1969). *J Gerontol*, 24, 2

Society of Actuaries (1959). Build and blood pressure study, p.268 (Chicago: The Society of Actuaries)

Kannell, WB and Gordon, T. (1974). In Burland, WL, Samuel, PO and Yudkin, J. (eds). Obesity Symposium, p.24. (Edinburgh: Churchill Livingstone)

Royal College of General Practitioners' Oral Contraceptive Study. (1983). Incidence of arterial disease among oral contraceptive users. *J R Coll Gen Practit*, 33, 75–82

Hodgson, JL and Buskirk, ER. (1981). Role of exercise in aging. In Danon, D, Shock, NW and Marois, M (eds) Ageing: a challenge to science and society, Vol.1, Biology, (Oxford University Press)

Section 3
Common Clinical Problems

ANOREXIA AND NUTRITIONAL PROBLEMS

Anorexia, when presented as an isolated symptom, strikes the general practitioner as ominous. Usually, however, associated pallor, jaundice, or mental change will be present. Features of undernutrition are:

> Mental dullness,
> Apathy
> Withdrawal,
> Muscular weakness,
> Changes in skin and mucous membranes,
> Anaemia,
> Low serum albumin,
> Low blood vitamin levels.

Where adequate food is available and there are no problems of absorption or utilization, there are three principal causes:

> Rejection of food,
> Unbalanced intake with adequate calories,
> Mechanical eating problems (dental, neurological, etc.).

Eating is a variable aspect of human behaviour. For many, the enjoyment of food is the one remaining pleasure, and one overindulged. Others, who have never been particularly interested, may eat within a narrow monotonous range. What is meant by anorexia must, therefore, bear some relation to individual norms.

A patient may find making a 24-hour recall of intake difficult, but a pattern of eating and an impression of kinds and amounts of food are more easily obtained. Since loss of appetite is often associated with changes in behaviour, mental state and energy output may be provided by a third party who knows the patient well. This information is important in assessing the calorific requirements for maintaining body weight which is the most important single observation for the assessment of nutritional status. Remember that weight loss may be due to fluid changes, but if it is due to loss of lean body mass it is accompanied by very little fat in the skinfolds.

This is a problem with many factors to consider. It is important to remember that dyspnoea can be a limiting factor in eating. Occasionally, a delusional state occurs when the patient believes that food is being poisoned.

Table 3.1 Causes of anorexia

	Common causes	Uncommon causes
Gastrointestinal	oral/dental dis. carcinoma	gastritis atrophic (P.A.) chronic alcohol abuse hepatic dysfunction pancreatic/biliary constipation
Functional/ psychiatric	depression dementia	anxiety delusion manipulation tremor
Social	isolation mobility problem self-neglect faddism	primary dietary disease Diogenes syndrome
Metabolic		uraemia dehydration hypothyroidism
Drugs	digitalis especially	

Dysphagia

This, occurring for the first time in later life, must be regarded with gravity. A few questions are important, beginning with the level at which obstruction is felt. In the upper third, or lower part of the chest, the likely cause is pharyngo-oesophageal obstruction, but it may also be due to neuromuscular inco-ordination, as occurs in bulbar and pseudo-bulbar palsy, diverticulae, and laryngeal or cervical tumours.

In the centre of the chest, the diagnosis is much more likely to be carcinoma of the oesophagus, or its compression by mediastinal lymph nodes, or an aortic enlargement, either aneurysm or an unfolded arteriosclerotic aorta. Where it is localized to the lower part of the chest, then the possibility of hiatus hernia arises, or a neoplasm of the oesophagus or stomach. Where dysphagia is present, enquiry should be made about whether the patient can swallow solid, or only liquid, food but each case must be investigated immediately, in the first place with a barium swallow or chest X-ray.

Weight loss

Loss of weight must be considered as important in the old as in the young. Before embarking on detailed investigation, make certain that the patient has in fact lost weight! This is not always easy but can sometimes be estimated by direct observation of poorly fitting clothes or lax skin folds. Some patients can remember their usual weight but, of course, it is usual for weight to increase with age, to plateau between 65 and 74, and then to fall for reasons which are obscure. In advanced age, a selective atrophy of depot fat begins at the periphery, and is more marked in women than in men, so weight loss in the trunk is nearly always significant.

Points to note in the history

- Has the patient really lost weight?
- Ask about the appetite.
- Is the nutritional state adequate?
- What do meals consist of?
- Where is food purchased and how is it cooked?
- Does the patient drink alcohol or smoke tobacco?
- Is there any difficulty or discomfort involved in swallowing food?
- Enquire about changes in bowel habit and the nature of stools.
- Does the patient have any other illness or take any drugs?
- Assess the mental state, memory, anxiety, depression, etc.
- Does the patient eat alone or in a club? Enquire about spouse and visits from relatives or neighbours.
- Ask about socio-economic factors – how much is spent on food and how near are the shops, etc?

It is easiest to consider weight loss in three broad categories:

1.   Normal appetite and adequate nutritional intake:

The pathology for weight loss in these circumstances include:

  malabsorption,
  excessive utilization,
  excessive loss.

Malabsorption may be due to the fact the mucosal surface of the small intestine tends to decrease with advancing age due to changes in the villi and mesenteric ischaemia. Abdominal scars may be scarcely visible and need searching for, but are important as indications of surgical intervention long ago, particularly partial gastrectomy or small bowel resection. Duodenal and other small bowel diverticulae may be colonized by abnormal commensals which absorb essential nutrients such as cyanocobalamin. Steatorrhoea may be due to benign disease of the pancreas, but is often idiopathic. Malabsorption may arise from carcinoma of the pancreas, but is sometimes found in association with conditions such as amyloidosis, scleroderma, diabetes, rheumatoid disease and neoplastic lesions. It can also result from the abuse of laxatives, although this is now less common than formerly.

Excessive utilization occurs when the tissues are used to provide energy in catabolic states. In a group practice covering 10,000 patients, GPs might expect to have one or two patients over the age of 65 with thyrotoxicosis, a disease which is commoner in women than men in a ratio of at least four to one. Remember also that the symptomatology is often atypical in older people, so that overactivity may give way to lethargic apathy and a syndrome of failure to thrive. Heart failure and atrial fibrillation resistant to therapy, restless sleep and altered mental function are important pointers to the diagnosis. It is important to review thyroid replacement therapy at regular intervals in order to determine if it is still necessary.

Excessive weight loss may be due to diabetes. The calorie loss resulting from glycosuria may be of the order of 100 g daily, and the weight loss is usually insidious. In ulcerative colitis and in regional ileitis, there may be a protein-losing enteropathy, but large amounts of protein loss from the kidneys is rare. Substantial losses may occur in expectoration from chronic lung disease, and exudation from large chronic ulcers and pressure sores. Finally, intestinal parasites must also be considered.

2. *Good appetite and inadequate nutritional intake:*

Here it is necessary to consider the physical, mental and social function of the patient. Those with impaired mobility are at a great disadvantage, and the complexity of the skills needed to carry out the normal activities of daily living are appreciated only once they are lost! Those elderly people who are independent and mobile within the house through the use of walking aids nevertheless find it virtually impossible to carry a hot meal or beverage. Unfortunately, the type of adaptation most frequently encountered is a reduction in the range of food, and a reliance on convenience foods of dubious nutritional value. Where there is impaired mental function, the inevitable result is self-neglect, while many over the age of 75 have only rudimentary ideas of nutritional requirements for good health. Some old people are at the mercy of unscrupulous shopkeepers in money matters.

3. Diminished appetite and inadequate nutritional intake

Most commonly, this is encountered as the result of psychogenic causes, and maybe due to excessive alcohol consumption and tobacco smoking, depression, or anxiety. Somatic causes must not be overlooked, such as chronic infections, renal failure, cardiorespiratory insufficiency and neoplastic lesions, the whole range of GI tract disorders, and rarities, such as Addison's disease and hypopituitarism.

Points to notice in the physical examination

- General appearance – wasting, cachexia, fit of clothes, loose skin folds, pigmentation.
- Specific signs – cheilosis, angular stomatitis, nasolabial seborrhoea, glossitis, spooning of nails, follicular haemorrhages, circumcorneal vascularization, fistula formation, etc.
- Abdomen – scars, masses, hepatic enlargement.
- Rectal examination
- Vaginal examination
- Systematic clinical examination

Investigations

The following list can be used selectively in accordance with the physical findings:

Complete blood picture and ESR,
Serum electrolytes,
Blood urea,
Creatinine,
Calcium,
Phosphate,
Alkaline phosphatase,
Albumin,
Total protein,
Protein electrophoresis,
Random blood glucose/GTT,

Serum thyroxine/tri-iodothyronine, TSH,
Stool – occult blood, ova and parasites,
If lesion in GI tract is suspected: sigmoidoscopy, Ba enema, Ba meal, gastroscopy

LOSS OF ENERGY AND THE COMPLAINT OF FATIGUE

Features of tiredness correspond to the culturally accepted pattern of senescence. Fatigue is a poorly understood phenomenon, implying abnormally rapid dissipation of energy during effort. Subjective impressions of the hardness of work actually correlate less with ergonomic measurements of work done than with rates of oxygen consumption and the effects of acidosis on the brain. Some old people's complaints are social, conventional and imaginary, having been conditioned to pursue life-styles of passivity, aimlessness, and guardianship. Thus, many factors contribute to the symptom of fatigue.

There is a vast number of factors to consider here – iatrogenic, deficiency states, chronic infections, and neurological and cardiorespiratory conditions. It is best, therefore, to consider, first the weight of psychological factors, the length of the history, the time of onset and the progression. Does the patient always feel fatigued, even after a full night's sleep? If so, psychological causes are most likely. Anxiety, boredom and depression may all be apparent in the manner of the patient's delivery and from the discussion of daily activities, the amount of sleep, its quality, the amount of food intake, and retained interests.

Because of the numerous contributions to the symptom, clinical examination must be thorough, and much may be gained from observing signs of neglect, cachexia, the corners of the mouth and the gait, in the general examination. It is important to see the patient perform some simple exercise, such as sitting up several times in order to see whether a triple or gallop rhythm is produced. A resting tachycardia is an important observation. Measure the respiratory rate at rest, check for enlarged lymph nodes in the neck, and inspect the superficial veins for signs suggesting raised venous pressure indicating congestive cardiac failure or observation of the mediastinum or the portal veins or vena cava. Skin lesions such as acanthosis nigricans and spider naevi are important indicators of general disease.

If the clinical examination is satisfactory, test results are normal, and the patient is not taking any medication that might be contributory, then he can be firmly reassured about the absence of disease, but should be seen again after three months. The days have long since gone when iron or a 'tonic' was given.

SLEEP DISORDERS AND INSOMNIA

The problem of insomnia, with the uneasy negotiations with old people and their relatives who have become unable to contemplate a night without regular hypnotic drugs, is one of the most contentious situations in general practice, particularly as the GP may not always have initiated the sleeping tablet ritual. It is strange that old people often attribute genuine disease to getting old, but still expect to maintain the same sleep pattern of earlier years.

There are many age changes in sleep, the major one being that the regular pattern of a full night's sleep is fragmented, and subject to frequent awakenings (a mean of 7.7 as against 2 in the young), but sleeping time lost is usually compensated for by periods of sleep taken during the day, meaning, in effect, that most old people get the same amount of sleep in the 24 hours as they did before.

Getting off to sleep takes longer, rising from 10 minutes on average in youth to 25 minutes over the age of 70. The duration of stage one sleep is usually prolonged, but the duration of stage four is often shorter and may be completely absent. The total period of REM sleep is not significantly altered, but, unlike younger people, it occurs early in the night and tends to become shorter as the night progresses. However, it remains a fact that healthy elderly people rarely regard sleep as a problem, which raises the question as to whether these changes are really due to ageing per se or to some other factor interfering with the sleep pattern.

There are about four times the number of complaints made about difficulty in falling asleep in people over 70 years of age compared with those aged 20, and twice as many complaints made by the elderly about difficulties experienced in maintaining sleep. It is not surprising, therefore, to learn that the elderly population consumes about 39% of all hypnotic preparations, and 15% of men and 30% of women are regularly taking such preparations.

Attitudes to sleep

A common lay belief persists that old people need more sleep when old and 'tired'. It is reinforced when they see old people dropping off in armchairs during the afternoon, and it never occurs to them that this might be due to boredom, postprandial insulin changes, or early signs of diseases such as uraemia. Neither does it seem to occur to many relatives that, having been put to bed early, an elderly person cannot sustain sleep during the night for long without waking, whether or not they suffer from the consequence of physical and mental discomforts, nor that there is a strong link between reversed sleep rhythm, wandering and obstreperous behaviour and the widespread tendency to take sedative drugs. It is quite common to find people taking any tablet lying to hand, such as an aspirin, and to sleep from the placebo effect! In any case, it is well known that sleep is the most unreliable testimony given in the history.

Common causes of sleep disorder

These multiply with age from a variety of causes such as pruritis, pain, angina, dyspnoea, and so on. Between the ages of 60 and 64, one male in four needs to rise and pass water at night – a figure that rises to more than 90% in the very old. In non-obese women, the rate is higher, but the rate of increase is less rapid, reaching only 83% in the 85 to 89-year-olds. Leg cramps affect 7% of the young elderly, but this is trebled after 15 years.

Palpitation, nocturnal angina and paroxysmal dyspnoea are not only physically disturbing, but create secondary anxiety. Cough and discomfort from LVF, or reabsorption of oedema fluid from the interstitial space, are sometimes confused with chronic chest diseases. It must be remembered that asthma is more common in the elderly than is generally believed. Pain from an ulcer or intestinal disorder may disturb sleep, as may hunger or hypoglycaemia. Psychological factors, such as fear, anxiety, depression and bereavement, are more commonly found in older age groups commonly believed to have reached a peaceful disengagement from life's problems!

Review of the drug list

Always review this, since drugs such as adrenergic agents may produce sympathetic stimulation, and beta-blockers can cause nightmares. Prescribed drugs may sometimes be obtained from other sources, so always ask specifically about this. Patients remain ignorant of the power of socially accepted beverages to produce insomnia, e.g. tea, whereas alcohol, a central depressant, can produce initial drowsiness and induce sleep, from which the sleeper later wakens and becomes restless, needing to urinate.

Physical conditions affect people less in their own homes than in nursing homes and other institutional settings, and, even when staying with relatives, such factors as noise, light, heat and humidity should be reviewed.

To prescribe or not to prescribe

This will depend very largely on the quality of the doctor/patient relationship, and whether sleeping tablets have previously been taken. Irritability and restless anxiety may follow withdrawal. Everything will depend on the sort of patient – whether they still drive, or whether they easily become habituated to drugs, with a vulnerable personality. The GP should soon be able to tell if the patient is responsive to advice about going to bed only when sleepy and avoiding cat naps during the day. He will also remember that CNS depressants are contraindicated in respiratory failure, and point out that he does not wish to blunt awareness to the presence of a full bladder in the night. He might even warn of the dangers of falls as a risk to those who need to make a journey at night to the toilet.

If a drug is to be prescribed, it should be on the understanding that, like an antibiotic, it is to be taken for a short time only. It should be selected from a short list of drugs which have a short half-life.

A practical approach to sleep disorders

- Define the precise nature of the problem.
- What does the patient mean by insomnia?
- What are the patient's expectations and fears concerning sleep?
- What is the 24-hour sleep pattern? (Include daytime naps, early waking, interruption.)
- What was the habitual sleep pattern? When did this change?
- What attempts have been made to restore it? (Include drugs prescribed and self-administered substances, e.g. alcohol, aspirin, tea.)
- Is the patient depressed, apathetic, agitated, demented?
- Perform a clinical examination, noting obesity, thyroid disorder, arthritis/mobility, oedema, hypertension, ischaemic heart disease, peripheral vascular insufficiency, chest disease, a full bladder or loaded rectum.

— Perform simple routine tests, such as routine blood and urine testing and ECG, and other tests depending on findings.

HEADACHE

Old people complain less of headache, but, when they do, it is of more sinister significance. By the mid-sixties, migraine as a cause of headache has virtually disappeared, perhaps due to hardening of the arteries. Instead, unilateral headache must be thought of as primarily due to cranial arteritis, unless proved otherwise. Tension headache, so common in the young, is almost never found in the old, perhaps due to reduction of muscle tone in the occipitofrontalis. However, occipital pain is not uncommonly associated with cervical spondylosis by strain imposed on the nuchal ligament through stooping posture.

Severe periodic headache, particularly where there has been a history of trauma and a rapid increase of symptoms for two to three weeks following injury, must lead one to consider a space-occupying lesion, in particular that of subdural haematoma. In this condition, the rapid increase in symptoms is due to lysis of red cells setting up an osmotic gradient across the arachnoid membrane. The occurrence of paralysis and periodic confusion may be mistaken tragically for incipient stroke, in which case the patient may be left at home and not offered surgery.

Check list of causes of headache in the elderly

Extracranial	*Intracranial*
Cervical spondylosis	Subdural haematoma
Cranial arteritis	Meningitis
Ocular disease	Abscess
Tic douloureux	Subarrachnoid haemorrhage
Cranial	Tumour
Diseases of the skull	General
e.g. Paget's	Fever
Dental	Phaeochromocytoma
Sinusitis	Carbon monoxide poisoning
Trauma	Depression
Otitis	Anxiety and tension
Glaucoma	Nephritis

DIZZY TURNS AND UNSTEADINESS

The problem of instability in an elderly patient is often puzzling, and it is often difficult to know how best to approach it. As many as half the over 70's suffer from dizziness, but it is a symptom that should always be taken seriously, as the resultant fall can lead to a total loss of confidence and even lead to the patient becoming bedridden. Complaints of dizziness are made between the ages of 65 and 80 with a marked female predominance. In both sexes, the incidence of accidental falls rises sharply between ages 65 and 85, and there is a rough division into those produced by intrinsic factors and those resulting from environmental hazards. The incidence of fractures also rises markedly over the age of 75. It is not enough to examine the patient who has fallen for signs of injury and shock, but the underlying causes must be sought in order to prevent recurrence.

The innumerable causes of dizziness are conveniently divided into two main groups.

Labyrinthine and CNS abnormalities

Disturbances in the labyrinth may be distinguished by the presence of nystagmus, while wax in the ear usually produces a feeling of unsteadiness rather than vertigo.

Circulatory and metabolic disorders

These can be considered in three areas:

> Supratentorial,
> Infratentorial,
> Cerebellopontine angle.

The most common infratentorial cause is vertebrobasilar insufficiency, while supratentorial lesions include epilepsy, psychogenic disorders and syncope.

At the cerebellopontine angle, bear in mind rarities, such as Paget's disease which produces abnormalities at the base of the skull, and also metastatic carcinoma.

The most common cause in practice is vertebrobasilar insufficiency provoked by sudden head movement, especially at the extremes, so that this can be tested for easily in the consulting room. However, it is in-

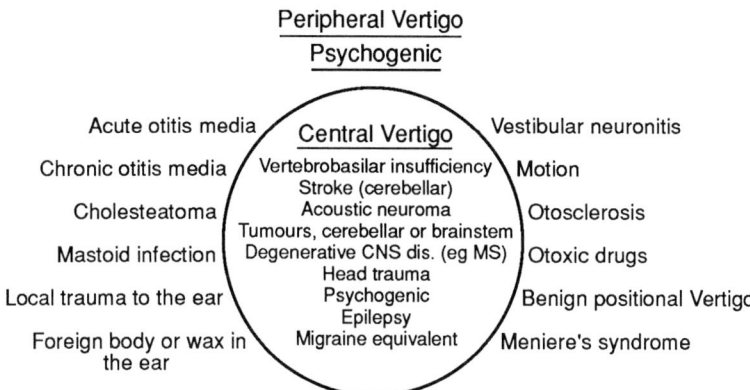

Figure 3.1 Causes of vertigo

creasingly recognized that older patients, particularly females, suffer from the sudden onset of cardiac tachyarrhythmias which reduce the cerebral blood flow temporarily, and may require detection by 24-hour ECG monitoring. Nor must it be overlooked that many somatic and social equilibria are upset in old age, and anxiety and the manifestations of chronic hyperventilation are responsible in some instances, together with the effects of memory impairment and visual disturbance (Figure 3.1).

In the management of vertigo, the most important function is an adequate examination, followed by a full explanation and strong reassurance, since, in most patients who suffer from vertigo, there is a natural tendency towards spontaneous resolution. This may be reinforced by advice to avoid excessive eating, drinking, smoking and head movements.

FALLING IN THE ELDERLY

The first thing to ascertain when taking the history is whether the fall was related to posture, e.g. on standing up, during exertion, or on moving the neck. This will direct the attention to postural hypotension, measured effectively by taking the blood pressure sitting and standing, or an inadequate cardiac output, as in aortic stenosis, or a sensitive carotid sinus or vertebrobasilar insufficiency. All these are preceded by a feeling of dizziness.

When a change of posture did not precede the fall, but dizziness was experienced, the association with tinnitus and deafness must be noted, and focal neurological deficit suspected.

Drop attacks, often mentioned, are quite rare in practice, but have to be considered. Although the drop attack is something from which the patient recovers spontaneously as a rule, it is important to remember that the fall itself may produce a head injury.

Investigations should normally include an ECG. The 12-lead ECG may show several arrythmias which predispose to falls, and a rhythm strip is important. During the latter, note the effect on the heart rate of carotid sinus compression. In certain cases, the only way to obtain the essentialk information is to refer the patient for 24-hour ambulatory ECG monitoring. Other important investigations include:

- X-ray of cervical spine for spondylosis,
- CXR, particularly for heart size,
- ESR anf full blood count – may indicate forms of arteritis or malignancy, or departures from the normal which increase heart load,
- Thyroid function tests may indicate a reason for proximal myopathy or atrial fibrillation,
- Serum electrolytes,
- Alkaline phosphatase,
- Random blood sugar.

Points to remember when examining someone who has fallen

Increased sway – with advancing age the ability to retain control of vertical posture declines, and self-righting reflexes become slower.

Arthropathies – unstable joints, muscle atrophy and straining to rise (Valsalva manoeuvre, e.g. in micturition syncope) all tend to produce falling.

Myopathies associated with thyrotoxicosis, Cushing's disease and osteomalacia and less common myopathies may be found.

Parkinson's disease may present with falling in the early stages.

Peripheral neuropathy from various causes: B_{12} deficiency, diabetes, chronic alcoholism, Guillain–Barré and other rare syndromes.

Cerebellar deficit and mental impairment.

Poor perception of the environment and visual impairment.

Environmental hazards, loose carpets, poor lighting, slippery bath, trailing wires, etc.

Drugs, prescribed or self-administered.

Signs of head injury, cardiac arrhythmia, new glasses (bifocals), foot problems, carotid bruits, mental status, blood pressure.

SIGHT AND HEARING

The doctor with an average practice will refer more problems concerning the special senses than to any other speciality. Even so, defects in the special senses often pass unnoticed unless sought for. Even when patients ask the doctor to repeat his question with hand cupped to ear, and everything should stop to ensure that the lines of communication are clear, doctors very often continue their original line of enquiry, for deafness remains an acceptable part of the picture of growing old, even to doctors. The onset of functional loss is so slow that patients adapt to the process, and do not complain. It is worth stressing that inefficiency due to age begins with changes in the sensory mechanism of the nervous system and its connections. The loss of stimulation thus suffered produces mental dulling, apathy, confusional or paranoid states, which can affect social mobility as effectively as hemiplegia or deforming arthritis, throwing the individual back on learned behaviour and ritual.

Vision and age changes

There is a much greater need in modern society for good visual capacity. Old people are busier than in former generations, but activities such as reading, watching theatrical and sporting performances, and TV, assume greater importance when retired. Only exceptional individuals retain normal visual activity in very old age: losses of acuity and colour vision are to be expected, connected with lenticular yellowing and physiological miosis. The amount of light reaching the retina is much less at 70 than it was at 20.

The most common external eye problems are due to lid changes producing entropion and ectropion, which should be dealt with before corneal damage has occurred. Dry eyes are more common, and cat lovers and keen gardeners need to be warned of the possibility of corneal damage from claws and sprays.

Ageing and vision

Numerous physiological changes take place in the ageing eye, the most important of which are presbyopia and physiological miosis which reduces the amount of light received by the retina. Other changes in the shape of the eye and its coverings, such as senile entropion, may threaten the integrity of the cornea, to say nothing of fondling cats which may scratch and spraying fruit trees without protective glasses. Conditions such as diminished tear production, herpes zoster ophthalmicus and ocular muscle paralyses are also more prevalent.

Visual deterioration late in life is important, not only because of loss of interest in the environment and consequent social withdrawal and depression, but because, unlike younger patients, new skills, such as wearing contact lenses and reading Braille, are difficult to attain. Routine examination of the eyes in people over 50 is therefore recommended.

Extraocular causes of visual impairment

Patients often persist in changing their glasses in the hope of seeing better, while others are found to be wearing spectacles which were prescribed for a visual state which has long since changed. In neglected patients, this may be confounded by the accumulated grease and dirt from handling, and much improvement can be made by cleaning the lenses in washing-up liquid! While the prescription for glasses frequently changes in women past the menopause, the urine should be tested whenever deteriorating vision is encountered since declining visual acuity may be the only apparent symptom of diabetic eye disease.

In giant cell arteritis, it is important to remember that headaches are present in only half the patients with this condition, while about a quarter are affected with blindness. Since giant cell arteritis may present without headache, but with general malaise, anorexia and weight loss, the family doctor must retain a high index of suspicion of this condition developing in the vaguely ill. The ESR is not always very high, but may lie in a moderate range that some GPs regard as normal for elderly people.

In the elderly, consideration has to be given to a wide range of vascular thrombotic and embolic occurrences, resulting from intracranial pressure, hypoxic hypercapnoea and drug effects.

Ocular causes of visual impairment

Over the age of 65, cataract is present in more than 90% of people, so that all patients should be screened by using the + 10 lens of the ophthalmoscope, when wedge-shaped spoke-like opacities or central nuclear dark areas are observed. The rate of advance is slow, and one eye is always affected before the other. There is no longer any need to wait for 'ripeness' before considering cataract extraction, which is now a very safe operation, though the number of those in whom the process becomes advanced enough to cause significant visual disability is small. The chief factor governing the decision to operate on an elderly individual is the functional integrity of the retina. Patients may need postoperative guidance if they find vision in the corrected aphakic eye enlarged and very brilliant, or contraction of the visual field with blurred contours outside the visual axis when aphakic glasses are worn. This is important for drivers, who now have to turn their heads through a right angle to survey traffic at cross roads. Increasingly now these difficulties are avoided by intraocular lens replacement.

On average, a case of acute closed angle glaucoma will occur once in 10 years in the practice, but will not be missed because of its dramatic onset. Primary glaucoma presents formidable difficulty as there are no early symptoms, and, by the time they show, retinal damage is irreversible. The family doctor should pay particular attention where there is a history of glaucoma in first degree relatives, but there is, of course, an increase in all types as age advances, simple open angle glaucoma being about four times more common than the closed angle type. Individual eyes vary in their ability to withstand a raised pressure without sustaining damage. Little reliance can be placed on the time-honoured method of confrontation to demonstrate field defects. Treatment of chronic simple glaucoma is usually by use of a beta-adrenoceptor drug, such as timolol maleate, which reduces intraocular pressure by reducing the rate of production of aqueous humour.

In angle-closure glaucoma, warning symptoms are pain around the eyes after reading, periodic blurring of vision, and coloured haloes seen around objects and lights. The optic disc may be abnormally cupped right to the edge, which is different from physiological cupping. Diurnal pressure changes are highest late at night, due to dilatation of the pupil. Avoidance of ingestion of large volumes of fluid, such as beer in the evening, is important, while long-term steroid therapy is an added risk. Management here is surgical, and primary angle closure is a bilateral disease. Care must be observed in prescribing anticholinergic drugs, including levodopa, tricyclic antidepressants and betamethasone.

Vascular occlusion

As a rule, vision is not completely lost in venous occlusion, and loss occurs more slowly than when the artery is occluded. Prognosis is poor. It may indicate the presence of a more general disease, such as proteinopathy. Occlusion of the central artery of the retina causes total blindness, and the macula stands out as a cherry-red spot. An embolus in a branch may sometimes be seen and may be moved suddenly by eye massage, breathing into a paper bag, or by IV injection of dipyridamole.

Macular degeneration

This is not uncommon, and is most often bilateral, affecting the macular portion of the retina, so that peripheral vision often remains intact, allowing one to reassure the patient that vision will never be completely lost. Patients do not look straight at you, but across your shoulder, as they employ their peripheral vision. Recognized early, photocoagulation may be employed – if not, all one can offer is the provision of visual aids.

Ageing and hearing loss

The frequency spectrum needed for understanding speech lies between 500 and 2000 Hz, and is not affected at first, but distortion due to loss of higher frequency occurs later, causing inability to distinguish the consonants in speech flow. It is wrong to imagine that hearing loss results only from loss in a specialized input sensory system, for it is a complex function involving neural pathways in the brain as well as cortical function. It is best to approach hearing problems in old people, therefore, without preconceptions, and to evaluate their hearing in terms of four areas:

1. The transformer

There is no evidence that senile changes in the ear drum contribute to hearing loss, although the drum often appears thicker and more opaque. Sound is mechanically transformed by the pinna, the canal, the tympanum and the middle ear with its pressure chamber and ossicles. The transformer ratio of 20:1 represents the difference in the area of the tympanic membrane and the stapedial area. Middle-ear defects essentially cause loss of volume.

2. The transducer

The mechanical energy of sound is converted in the cochlea by hair cells of the organ of Corti, high-tone reduction occurring through loss of cells towards the base. Many factors lead to this, including autosomal dominant progressive hearing loss which make genetic enquiries important. Environmental noise and other conditions, such as ototoxic drugs (especially aspirin), should be enquired about.

3. The connector

The eighth nerve is subject to several types of disease in the elderly, the most important being acoustic neuroma.

4. The analyser

The central nervous system acts as the end station in the hearing pathway, and elderly people have more difficulty in understanding language than might be suspected from studying their pure tone audiograms.

Bear in mind that hearing problems in the middle ear resemble those in earlier life, but that infection as the most common cause may be related to diabetes or Paget's disease, for which new drugs are becoming available. Wax is more likely to impact, and, because of thinning, the skin lining the canal becomes more delicate and liable to infection.

If hearing loss is predominantly in the middle ear, and not due to infection, surgical correction should be considered.

Lesions of the inner ear, if not too extensive, can be greatly helped by the proper use of hearing aids.

Severe and total loss of hearing can be helped by training in lip reading.

For some reason, we have less patience with the deaf than with the blind, and there is an important association between deafness and paranoid psychosis. Social isolation can occur, even within the family. Help is obtainable from the RNID, who will send synopses of certain programmes on TV to the very deaf, who can also benefit from Ceefax 888 subtitles.

Hearing aids are simply amplifying systems, and old people need protection against excessive claims by doorstep salesmen. Those worn at ear level have the advantage that the aid can turn with the head towards the sound source, and there is elimination of noise from the friction of clothing. Above all, it is more acceptable psychologically. Such aids can be worn behind the ear or built into the frames of glasses. They have equivalent performance characteristics of up to about 50 dB of useable gain.

Binaural aids improve localization of sound and lead to better speech intelligibility against background noise. All aids need to be regularly checked.

DYSPNOEA ON EXERTION

Old people get used to living within the limits imposed by a limited respiratory reserve capacity. However, the threshold at which dyspnoea is experienced from other causes is lowered. So, mild infections may reduce a patient's capacity for effort quite markedly. Smoking may seriously reduce performance where there is impaired perfusion capacity. Arterial oxygen pressure is much lower than in the young so confusion and brain anoxia threaten the patient who develops pulmonary infection. There are no specific ECG changes with ageing, but changes in the heart due to age are numerous.

In the history, attention is paid to features such as sudden onset and consistency of distress to the same amount of effort.

Chronic bronchitis is incompatible with advanced age, but is not always associated with smoking. Superinfection occurs in autumn and winter, and patients may be given a small starting dose of a broad spectrum antibiotic, and should be immunized against prevalent strains of influenza shortly after the autumn equinox. Bronchial asthma is more common than generally believed, but, unlike chronic bronchitis, the PEF gives evidence of reversibility. Asthma patients tend to have their attacks at night with disturbed sleep, and are usually non-smokers.

Bronchial carcinoma ranks high among suspected diseases in the UK, but presentations vary and dyspnoea on exertion is not always the presenting complaint.

If emphysema develops in the senium, once the chest wall has become rigid the classic barrel-shaped chest described in most textbooks is presented.

Pulmonary hypertension and cor pulmonale are characterized by RVF, due more to severe hypoxia than obstruction to flow.

It is worth noting that warmth of the extremities is produced by hypercapnia, and is lost once heart failure sets in and peripheral vasoconstriction produces coldness.

Pulmonary emboli may also cause dyspnoea, gradually eroding the respiratory reserve capacity.

Spontaneous pneumothorax, as a result of punctured bullae, is not uncommon, and, characteristically, the chest is long and thin, but a small pneumothorax may be difficult to distinguish from emphysema. Pain is a feature, and an X-ray exposed at the end of expiration is diagnostic.

Cardiovascular causes

Myocardial ischaemia may become superimposed on poor cardiac reserves without pain sensation. Auscultation of the heart after exercise may enable triple rhythm to be detected. Choking and palpitation often accompany dyspnoea on exertion. Dyspnoea due to arrythmia is likely to occur where partial heart block is present, the degree of which may be increased by exertion. Arrythmia may arise at any time and the patient should be examined at rest since an elevated cardiac output then is suggestive of the altered haemodynamics due to thyrotoxicosis or anaemia.

It seems reasonable to reduce the load on a hypertrophied left ventricle by reducing blood pressure. Certain drugs, however, may produce dyspnoea on exertion, such as beta-blockers, digoxin, steroids and other anti-inflammatories, by slowing the heart, expanding the blood volume, or causing blood loss.

Obesity, of course, influences the heart/weight ratio but reduces thoracic compliances.

Table 3.2 A practical approach to dyspnoea on exertion

The history	Clinical appearance	Laboratory investigation
Mode of onset	General appearance:	Full blood count and ESR
Severity	obesity	Urine analysis
Daily activities &	plethora	Chest X-ray
physical exercise	cyanosis	Sputum examination
Duration and course	pallor	ECG
Associated symptoms:	clubbing	Lung function tests
palpitation	Rheumatoid disease	Blood culture (?infective
cough	Paget's (cardiac effect)	endocarditis)
nocturia	Cardiovascular system:	
orthopnoea	tachycardia	
oedema	bradycardia	
Smoking habits	pulsus bigeminus	
Previous occupations	atrial fibrillation	
Appetite	blood pressure, high or low	
Loss of weight	L.V. hypertrophy	
Any GI tract surgery	valvular lesions (?infective	
All medication	endocarditis)	
	triple rhythm	
	third heart sound	
	gallop rhythm	
	other signs of failure	
	Respiratory system:	
	shape of chest – kyphoscoliosis	
	deviation of trachea	
	tachypnoea	
	signs of lungs, e.g. hyper-resonance, wheeze	

Finally, dyspnoea may occasionally be due to anxiety and psychogenic causes, but, in this case, performance by the patient is not consistent.

Congestive cardiac failure

CCF is quite commonly encountered in the ambulatory aged, in whom a single cause is rarely responsible, although ischaemic and hypertensive heart disease predominate. Consider, therefore, the role of extra cardiac causes, such as anaemia, anoxia, thyrotoxicosis, and, rarely, Parkinson's disease, Paget's disease and thiamine deficiency.

Diagnosis

This is not always easy in the elderly since there may be mental confusion superimposed, difficulty in hearing heart sounds, and oedema from non-cardiac causes. Breathlessness, which may be confused with dyspnoea, may arise from obesity, emphysema, or a generally reduced ventilatory capacity which develops in advanced age. Enquire about orthopnoea, for this provides a better indication of failure. Remember that the presence of oedema in the ankles may be due to nothing more than dependency or venous stasis: so do not treat oedema as such with diuretic drugs. Be alert to early symptoms, such as nocturnal cough and wheezing, increased fatigability, angina, and insomnia associated with restlessness. A chest X-ray is helpful in showing cardiac enlargement and pulmonary congestion. It may also provide useful information about pulmonary infarction, emphysema and bronchitis. The ECG is valuable in helping to pinpoint the cause of heart failure. A normal tracing will indicate extra cardiac causes.

Rheumatic carditis is now working its way through the older age groups. Infective endocarditis, therefore, must be thought of and excluded, because its presentation is often atypical, with weight loss, pyrexia, mental confusion and a raised ESR, especially where a mitral murmur is present. In fact, it is easily mistaken for the caricature of 'old age coming on'. Remember that splinter haemorrhages in the nails are very rare and unreliable, because they may be produced by the grip of an aid while walking, so that they are more significant if found in the conjunctivae.

The variety of murmurs and their causes, arrhythmias and conduction disturbances, some only found on ECGs, make this an aspect of cardiology where specialist advice may readily be sought.

Management – Effective treatment in the elderly requires general measures that:

(1) Reduce the work of the heart,
(2) Prevent salt and water accumulation,
(3) Improve cardiac output.

Whole body rest is important in reducing heart rate and lengthening the diastolic interval, but the well-known dangers of bed-rest apply no less to cardiac patients. So, a suitable armchair with arms, in which the patient can sleep and from which he can rise easily, has considerable advantages. Some may benefit by spending a day in bed regularly each week. If prolonged rest is needed, the patient should be mobilized after one week. Failure in response during the first week is a grave sign. Attention should then be directed to eliminating and correcting extracardiac causes. Night time sedation may be needed for a short period, and thioridazine is useful for this purpose.

A recovered patient should be advised to climb stairs once a day and to stop frequently if distress arises. Visiting the home with the community nurse and health visitor is important in planning a treatment programme.

Drugs
Patients in sinus rhythm are best managed with thiazide or loop diuretics only. Standard potassium supplementation is no longer universally favoured, but potassium-sparing drugs may be used where lean body mass and total body potassium are proportionally reduced.

The GP should not fail to realize the social restrictions that these drugs can cause, and that facilities for passing urine must be readily accessible. It is not sensible to have the patient toiling upstairs a dozen times each morning to micturate. So, the decision to prescribe must be taken with proper planning. Some oedema may be tolerated, especially where the patient's activity is routine or circumscribed, such as in a home for the elderly. Oxygen and fluid intake should also be considered, for patients often reduce fluid intake in an attempt to reduce bothersome nocturia, while the sense of thirst as an indicator of dehydration is deficient in old people.

Digitalis has been used successfully for 200 years, but views on the indications for its use are changing. Its therapeutic margin is narrow, and it needs careful monitoring, checking the ventricular rate and ECG changes. It is most effective in cases of failure with atrial fibrillation and cardiomegaly. It is rarely needed for long-term therapy, although some patients deteriorate without it.

New drugs becoming important in the management of cardiac failure are the angiotensin-converting enzyme inhibitors, bringing about reduction in afterload by lowering systemic arteriolar resistance through vasodilatation. Drugs, such as captopril and enalapril, may be used in very small doses to begin with, after reduction of diuretic dosage. Such a procedure should be carried out under hospital conditions where close regular observation is possible.

BLOOD PRESSURE IN OLD AGE

At about 60 years of age, diastolic blood pressure tends to decrease but systolic pressure continues to rise, leading to an increase in pulse pressure (Figure 3.2). Body weight remains the main correlate of blood pressure level but this correlation between systolic and diastolic BP and obesity diminishes with age, and becomes negligible after the age of 60. High blood pressure is the main cardiovascular risk factor. Can we prevent blood pressure rising with age?

Arterial hypertension has few symptoms at any age, but high blood pressure may aggravate symptoms, such as vertigo, loss of balance or tinnintus, in the elderly. The treatment of hypertension should therefore aim to alleviate symptoms, if any, and improve general well being. it should reduce, or prevent, end-organ damage, and, in particular, reduce the incidence of myocardial infarction, stroke and other cardiovascular complications.

Each elderly patient poses an individual problem in respect of the blood pressure, and frequent measurements are desirable if one is to know

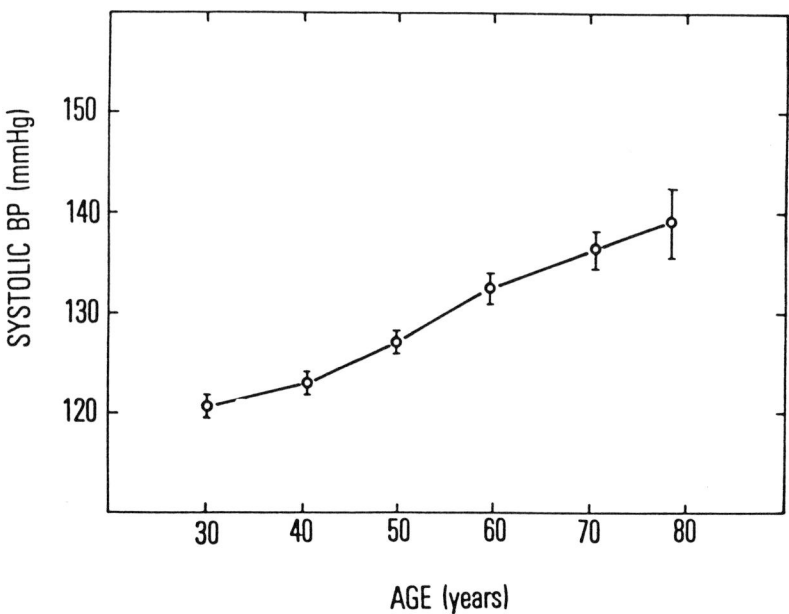

Figure 3.2 Effect of age on systolic blood-pressure. Clean group. The Ns for each decade from 30–80 were 82, 151, 184, 119, 103, and 35

what is happening. For instance, falling blood pressure is of serious import, heralding a failing heart, or metastasizing carcinoma, while rising blood pressure may indicate renal impairment or polyarteritis.

One's policy should probably be that high blood pressure should be controlled from middle age into old age, and continued then with the aim of preventing the otherwise inevitable complications of stroke, heart and renal failure. A time of particular danger for all hypertensives, particularly the elderly, is when there is transfer from one doctor to another. All such patients should have a bridging letter addressed to the new doctor to maintain continuity during the hiatus in the availability of medical records.

The regular finding of a blood pressure level of more than 170/95 in men and 190/75 in women should lead to thorough examination of heart size, state of the fundus, lung bases, and signs of organ damage.

The urine should be tested, and an ECG may be desirable since evidence of LV hypertrophy is an indication for treatment. A full blood count, fasting blood sugar, blood urea and electrolyte estimation is required if end organ damage is suspected, or before any intention to offer treatment.

Guiding principles for treating arterial hypertension

Each patient must be treated individually. To begin with, non-pharmacological means should be used to treat an elderly patient, even though it may be difficult to persuade him to change his habits. A decrease in salt intake, reduction of body weight, attention to the management of tension and anxiety, and mild exercise should be encouraged (although it is not known whether regular exercise lowers the blood pressure) as it increases the sense of well being. Relaxation therapy and bio-feedback are recently developed non-pharmacological treatments.

Drug treatment is commenced:

(1) When diastolic blood pressure repeatedly exceeds 100 mmHg (13.3 kPa),
(2) When the patient has complications associated with hypertension,
(3) When the patient's symptoms are related to high blood pressure.

As in younger individuals, beta-adrenergic receptor blocking agents or diuretics are the drugs of choice for beginning treatment in the elderly. Before prescribing beta-blockers, the possible contraindications should be investigated, but they often will be tolerated because they do not cause postural hypotension. The haemodynamic status of elderly patients being treated with beta-blockers must be carefully controlled as they are susceptible to congestive heart failure. The starting daily dose should therefore be half that for younger patients, and they should be watched closely in the initial phase of therapy, and after each increase in dose.

Thiazides are preferable to loop diuretics as they induce a more progressive and longer lasting diuresis, except for a patient whose renal function is impaired to such a degree that he has become unresponsive to any of the thiazides. Therapy should be started with a small dose, such as 2.5 mg bendrofluazide. Most thiazides are contraindicated in patients with gout and should be prescribed with care to those with diabetes mellitus. In the hypertensive patient with heart failure, a diuretic is particularly indicated.

If the hypotensive response is inadequate a beta-blocker may be added. Methyldopa has been used widely, and well tolerated, but it may cause drowsiness, depression, dryness of the mouth and orthostatic hypotension. It should not be prescribed for patients with liver damage.

In some elderly patients, it may be necessary to add a vasodilating agent, such as hydralazine, but this sometimes causes tachycardia. Experience with converting enzyme inhibitors, such as captopril and enalapril, suggests that captopril may be less effective in the elderly because of the age-related decrease in plasma renin activity. By contrast, the effectiveness of calcium antagonists, such as verapamil and nifedipine, may be greater in older than in younger patients.

Postural hypotension

Particular care needs to be taken to avoid postural hypotension, since hypotensive drugs are a leading cause of this potentially dangerous condition, leading to falls. Patients should be warned to rise slowly from bed to chairs. Most at risk are those also suffering from varicose veins, anaemia and hyponatraemia.

Chest pain

The diagnosis of chest pain in older patients is difficult, not only because the differential diagnosis is wide, but because pain is not simply present in only those with a condition, and absent in those without it.

In myocardial infarction, at least a third of infarcts are unrecognized because of this. Although they are five times more common in the over-60's than in the 40–49 age group, half these infarcts are 'silent'. The value of the chest X-ray cannot be stressed too strongly, for it is of greater diagnostic value than the ECG, differentiating other causes, such as pulmonary emboli and spontaneous pneumothorax, malignancy and mediastinal conditions.

Of the gastrointestinal causes of chest pain, reflux oesophagitis, with or without hiatus hernia, is the most difficult, and, in fact, the two conditions often co-exist. Relation to pain produced by recumbency after food intake is helpful, just as those arthritides which radiate into the chest become worse at night when joints, such as shoulder, now become weight-bearing. Also, acute abdominal conditions which sometimes mimic myocardial infarction may be differentiated by a past medical history. Psychosomatic chest pain is often related to deaths of a close friend or relative from ischaemic heart disease which has been witnessed.

Very occasionally, chest pain may be due to herpes zoster before the appearance of the rash.

Causes may therefore be cardiovascular, musculo-skeletal, respiratory, or abdominal in origin, as well as neurological or psychogenic.

The scheme in Table 3.3 may be helpful when chest pain does present.

BACK PAIN IN THE ELDERLY

The caricature of old age with a person stooped forward and walking with pain and difficulty, one hand holding the lower back, is more often seen in men in their thirties! However, while degenerative changes are inevitable with increased age, the spine also becomes more rigid, producing a splinting effect on movements that might produce pain. This results from osteophyte formation which may be gross enough to be mistaken for ankylosing spondylitis. Often asymptomatic, sometimes it causes persistent pain.

In the mobile regions of the spine, the cervical and lumbar regions are most likely to cause cord compression, and gross disc protrusion in the lumbar region may produce numbness, weakness and pain in one or both legs, known as claudication of the cauda equina.

Table 3.3 Presentations of chest pain according to site and character

Lower substernal (hiatus hernia) Worse lying flat or following meals, Aggravated by alcohol, Relieved by antacids, standing or walking.	*Central, poorly localized (angina)* Precipitated by exercise or emotion, Over-riding desire to stop activity, Duration 2–10 minutes, Rapid relief from GTN and rest, Referral to neck, lower jaw, shoulder, arm, back Variants: Prinzmetal, unstable, crescendo
Dull ache Nerve root compression, Sharp twinges superimposed, History of back pain, Tender spots Precipitated by movements of spine, incorrect posture, coughing, Relieved by rest.	*Severe crushing (myocardial infarction)* Not relieved by rest, Lasting more than 30 minutes Sweating, nausea, anxiety Often preceding episodes of discomfort.
Association with general muscular Systemic: polymyalgia rheumatica Polymyositis Dermatomysitis	*Sharp tearing (dissecting aneurysm)* Radiation according to pathway of dissection, Suspect when MI-type pain radiates to back.
Psychosomatic History of recent death with chest pain as marked feature of illness	*Persistent, localized* Pleuritic: worse on deep breathing Embolism; sudden dyspnoea, haemoptysis

Dorsal root pain is more common in the elderly, and this is produced by rotation phenomena: hyperaesthesia may be found around one side of the chest on stroking. The incidence of upper lumbar root compression, seen in younger age groups, rises sharply in later life. Despite abundant radiographic evidence of disc degeneration, erosion of apophyseal joints and osteoporosis in old people, this correlates poorly with symptoms.

Postural and degenerative changes cannot be separated. Poor sitting position, muscle weakness and the weight of the head, produce angulation of the neck on the lower spine. Pain is due to stretching of the ligaments about the intervertebral joints. The pain of spondylolisthesis is the same but localized.

Many other degenerative disorders contribute to back pain, such as osteoarthritis of the hips, Paget's disease, hemipareses and impacted femoral neck fractures. Pain is often produced by forward or backward stretching of the spine causing pain in ligaments already stretched to their limits.

Prolapse of intervertebral discs occurs more commonly in middle than in late age, but, in old people, discs are affected at levels higher than the usual L5/S1 site, and the X-ray report is often a catalogue of degeneration at several levels. It is important to interpret radiation into the lateral part of the leg as the result of compression of the fifth lumbar segment: instead of the customary loss of the ankle jerk, the knee jerk may be lost and the stability of the knee reduced when the fourth lumbar segment is compressed. Patients with multiple disc lesions may find it difficult to stand erect and may bend away from the painful side.

Osteoporosis is extremely common in thin women of N. European origin who smoke, but it is not painful until demineralization reaches the point where collapse occurs, usually just below a region of kyphosis, where unnatural forces are exerted. Osteoporosis is, of course, closely associated with the endocrine system, and the administration of corticosteroid drugs.

The angle of the sun in the British Isles from October to April is insufficient to produce vitamin D by radiation under the skin, and about 16% of the elderly female population of Scotland is thought to be affected by osteomalacia. This pain is a dull ache, not usually severe, but its inconstancy and vagueness easily suggest a neurotic complainer.

Paget's disease, though thought of in terms of larger hats, affects the weight-bearing bones more frequently than the rest of the skeleton, the pain being worse at night when the patient is warm.

Neoplastic lesions sometimes cause back pain, and, of the primary lesions, multiple myeloma is most common. But the prime suspects are secondary deposits: the prostate is always thought of in the elderly male; in both sexes, lung and kidney; and, in the female, the breast and thyroid.

Leriche's syndrome is where gradual occlusion of the lower end of the aorta and its bifurcation occurs, causing low back pain as well as poor blood flow to the limbs.

Low back pain may also result from an abdominal aortic aneurysm, retroperitoneal malignancies, chronic pancreatitis, as well as carcinoma of pancreas. Other causes in the elderly female include ovarian cyst, fibroid uterus, and, in either sex, renal pathology, such as calculus.

A good history is very important in sorting out, for example, sudden onset, nocturnal pain, radiation to the groin, the sex of the patient etc., coupled with good observation of the patient's appearance and clinical examination.

THE PAINFUL HIP JOINT

Be careful not to ascribe every painful hip to osteoarthritis, although it is the most common cause. If one does, remediable causes may be missed, so that one may be left with an elderly patient still complaining of difficulty in walking, after unsuccessful ingestion of anti-inflammatory analgesics, and even suffering from their complications!

Hip pain is often poorly localized, radiating to the knee, groin or medial thigh. Also, the pain of systemic diseases is often widespread, involving the hip, and nerve root compression will involve the hip and the back.

The pain in osteoarthritis is of slow evolution, usually affects one hip before the other, and tends to get worse as the day advances. In rheumatoid disease, the reverse is the case, and other joints are usually affected.

Sudden onset must alert one to the possibility of impacted femoral neck fracture, the history of trauma having been absent or forgotten. It is worth remembering that Paget's disease predisposes to osteosarcoma, while there are extra-articular causes in the various bursae around the hip, and acute calcific periarthritis.

Examination

The examination, beginning with inspection, should include measurement of each lower limb from the anterior superior iliac spine, simply because scoliosis may give a false impression of shortening.

The joint should be palpated for tenderness, local heat, and even swelling, since septic arthritis may still occur.

After measuring the range of passive movements, noting crepitus and muscle tone, upward pressure may be applied to the sole of the foot with the leg extended. This causes pain if there is an impacted fracture.

Finally the gait should be observed.

The diagnosis will be established by radiology, but it is worth mentioning on the request form that fracture may be present, so that X-rays may be taken from different angles. Occasionally, aspiration of the joint is carried out for examination of the fluid for crystals, cytology and organisms. A raised ESR may indicate polymyalgia rheumatica, rheumatoid disease or metastatic deposits.

Management

It seems that it will be Utopia when all who require surgery can receive it. For many years, the GP's role will be to maintain activity, and reduce pain and disability. Unfortunately, the part played by antirheumatic drugs in this condition is minor. The patient needs much reassurance as treatment is planned. While weight reduction may be insisted upon, it is achieved in only 5% of patients, largely due to restricted mobility. The provision of an inner sole to correct pelvic tilt is often helpful. A walking stick, correctly used, transfers 60% of the weight across from the painful hip, and is, perhaps, the most important recommendation. The most useful instrument I found in my surgery was a small saw to reduce the height of sticks used by shrunken women who came in carrying sticks formerly owned by a husband or brother. The stick should have a curved handle, and, when placed on the ground, should reach to the ulnar styloid. Attempts should be made to avoid stair climbing, and chair height should be increased, while arms assist the patient to rise. Referral to the physiotherapist will maintain morale and prevent atrophy of muscles.

SKIN IRRITATION

A common problem is itchy skin which appears to be normal, with no signs of rash or infestation. All that may be observed is a fine branny scaling, which is more common in winter, and is probably related to dehydration of the skin during spells when dry Arctic air affects the northern hemisphere for short periods.

The effect of age on the skin results in thinning and loss of appendages, sweat glands, etc. Patients should be advised to use a bath oil, and to avoid alkaline soaps which can produce maddening aggravation. After such a bath, the skin should be dabbed with a towel and left slightly moist while a light dressing gown is worn. Care must be taken, however, because oils make the bottom of the bath slippery, increasing the danger of falling.

Some people need only be advised to do this once a week, at other times, to sponge the intertriginous areas, applying a baby oil to the still moist skin.

Some people suffer badly when they are confined to bed in hot weather, due to occlusion of sweat glands and production of a form of miliaria. Here, cooling and improved ventilation is required. The affected skin can be soothed by thin spreading of ung. aqueous, or where there is inflammation, by using a steroid aerosol.

Not infrequently, one encounters patients, usually elderly females, with neurodermatitis of the nuchal region, seen as a pale discrete purplish area. This is maintained by scratching, and attention should be directed to breaking the vicious circle by using a steroid ointment and warning the patient not to scratch.

Another localized skin problem sometimes found in old people is delusional. They believe the skin has been invaded by parasites, and small rolls of epidermis may be saved for the doctor's visit as evidence of 'maggots' scratched from holes in the face. This is often associated with involutional depression or a paranoid type of dementia. One great difficulty is that relatives are also convinced when the story is told by a patient who has always enjoyed a reputation for telling the truth! Therapeutic management is very difficult, but one may try phenothiazine drugs with an innocuous cream for placebo effect. Above all, the practitioner must avoid confrontation by denial.

The physician will always have at the back of his mind, especially when pruritis is generalized, diseases such as malignancy, advanced liver disease, thyroid dysfunction, polycythaemia, gout, and adverse reactions to drugs. Symptomatic treatment may produce some relief, using those antihistamines which produce drowsiness and are effective for that reason only.

Previous history and past occupation may help to understand what is going on, as well as the personality of the patient, some of whom fear being considered 'dirty' in old age, and use soap and water excessively, producing fine mosaic fissuring of the skin.

It must be remembered, also, that, while most skin treatment can be carried out at home, the ability of old people to carry out a prescribed self-treatment may be greatly limited by poor vision, joint stiffness and mental change.

OEDEMA OF THE LOWER LIMBS

This is an excellent example of the situation where the patient should be considered as a whole. Events leading up to accumulation of fluid in the interstital space may result from increase in intracapillary hydrostatic pressure, changes which may, in turn, be dependent on the concentration of plasma protein in the vascular system, changes in capillary permeability produced by severe anoxia, and pressure effects dependent on the quality of venous return facilitated by the muscular contraction.

So far as aetiology is concerned, congestive cardiac failure affects both legs equally, as a rule, but the commonest type of oedema found in the elderly is postural or gravitational. This is more pronounced towards the end of the day and is usually quite soft. It is found in those with mobility problems, such as Parkinson's disease or hemiplegia, but most frequently in those who admit to spending most of the time sitting in a chair. Of course, heart disease and inactivity may be present together.

When due to deep venous thrombosis, oedema is usually asymmetrical, but the classical signs of DVT may not be present. The diagnosis may need to be confirmed by ultrasound when calf muscle compression fails to increase femoral vein blood flow.

Compression of pelvic veins, or the inferior vena cava by pelvic or intraabdominal masses produces oedema which is unilateral or bilateral, depending on the size of the mass and the way pressure is exerted.

It is important to realize that, in chronic bronchitis and emphysema, venous return to the heart is impeded, leading, not only to venous congestion, but to associated carbon dioxide retention, leading to capillary vasodilatation which may encourage exudation of fluid into the interstitial space.

Some other causes need to be considered in the elderly, such as diminished osmotic pressure due to hypoalbuminaemia in malnutrition, impaired synthesis in the liver, or excessive loss from the GI tract. The mechanism by which patients with hemiplegia often present with oedema of the paralysed side is not entirely understood, but is probably a result of alteration of autonomic nerve supply. In hypothyroid patients, it must be remembered that myxoedematous tissue accumulates in the interstital space and does not pit on pressure.

Management

Diuretics are of limited value in management of oedema of the lower limbs except when it is due to congestive cardiac failure. The effect of high-potency loop diuretics depends on there being free communication between the interstital and intravascular space.

If this communication is not free, or the mobilization of fluid from the interstital space is slow and does not match the increase in urine output produced, then central hypovolaemia results, diminishing the cardiac output and renal perfusion, so increasing renin production, increased angiotensin II, which in turn increases the output of aldosterone, stimulating reabsorption of salt and water from the renal tubules. In these circumstances, it would be better to prescribe a medium-potency or low-potency diuretic, or aldosterone antagonists where high-potency loop diuretics have been tried, producing excessive amounts of urine without reducing oedema.

Of course, diuretics cannot control gravitational or postural oedema of the lower limbs, for here mobilization is the important therapeutic measure. This may require pain control in arthritis or the treatment of Parkinsonism. If mobilization is not possible, isometric exercises are useful. Elastic bandages or stockings, used to control the hydrostatic pressure outside the vascular compartment, are useful providing care is taken to include the toes and avoid injuring the underlying skin. Thus, the rate of accumulation of fluid in the interstital space is reduced.

SHAKINESS AND TREMOR: AGEING OR DISEASE?

Older patients hardly ever complain of tremor directly. Therefore, it has to be looked for. There are four major diagnoses to be considered:

    Parkinson's disease,
    Senile tremor,
    Emotional tremor,
    Toxic tremor.

In Parkinson's disease, the disease develops insidiously and not all patients show tremor as a sign. However, it is often the presenting sign and is described as a 'pill-rolling' movement. It is not always present in early cases, which are usually unilateral, becoming more marked when the patient is engaged in conversation or is emotionally disturbed. Conversely, the tremor may disappear on performing a voluntary movement and is absent during sleep.

Senile tremor may be the same condition as benign essential or familial tremor, the tremor usually being finer and more rapid than that in Parkinson's disease, but, in some cases, coarser and slower. The main distinguishing feature is that, unlike Parkinsonian tremor, it is increased by voluntary movement and may be present, in the late stages, at rest.

Anxiety is common in the elderly and so is the phenomenon of disinhibition where emotional control is more tenuous. Anxiety and fear produce a tremor which is usually fine, but which may become coarse if hysteria occurs, although this shows a tendency to diminish when the patient is distracted.

The tremor of chronic alcoholism is fine, although that of delerium tremens is somewhat coarser. Other drugs are known to produce tremor, such as selective β_2-adrenoceptor stimulants, used in reversible airways obstruction, and others, when withdrawn, such as drugs of the diazepam series. Uncommonly, but to be borne in mind these days, is intoxication with cocaine.

A rare cause of tremor is cerebellar disease Static tremor develops if the patient attempts to keep the limb in the fixed position. Tremor on voluntary movement is partly due to faulty fixation and partly due to defective co-ordination which leads to a limb deviating first in one direction and then in another.

Thyrotoxicosis is a rare cause in old age, for it usually has monosystemic effects on the cardiovascular system, but, in a few patients, fine tremor of the outstretched hands may be found as a physical sign of this disease.

The recent increase in primary syphilis in some Western countries suggests that neurospyhilis is not a diagnosis to be shelved and may be seen again occurring 10–15 years after the initial infection, producing a coarse tremor of the hands, lips and tongue, and an Argyll–Robertson pupil associated with deterioration of the intellect with grandiose ideas. Unlike Parkinson's disease, the handwriting tends to be large and poorly controlled.

It must not be overlooked that some patients with multiple sclerosis survive into old age and are seen then after many years, or even for the first time. Flapping tremor, well-known as a feature of liver failure, may also be present in respiratory or renal failure.

In managing the tremulous patient, it is important to reassure those suffering from the quite common condition of senile tremor that their disorder is not due to the more progressive disorder of Parkinson's disease. It may also be worth pointing out that the condition is usually familial and is aggravated by stress and voluntary movement. The effect of the adrenergic component may be inhibited by β-blockade, but patients often find for themselves the beneficial effect of alcohol. It is, of course, unwise to suggest its use except on important social occasions, perhaps, such as a Golden Wedding when the glass raised to toast the spouse needs to be steady!

SEX PROBLEMS

The myth persists, even among practitioners, that old people are asexual beings. Many doctors find it embarrassing to ask about their sexual activities, although this is important, for instance, when referring a woman over 65 for a repair of uterine prolapse as the surgeon will need to tailor the operation accordingly. Of course, the sexual attitudes from Victorian times spread over into those born during the 1920's. The destructive social image of an old man who is healthy and retains a sexual appetite as a 'dirty old man' has led to an unfeeling attitude on the part of residential home administrators, and has made many old people abandon expressions of sexual need and interest for fear of ostracism, or even of being thought unnatural or dangerous!

In discussing sexual matters with the elderly, and often with their relatives, it must be realized that the origin of many problems lies in faulty training, low expectation, high inhibition, reduced opportunity, and the anxiety of society in general in regard to sexual matters.

Some facts

The effect of ageing on human sexual performance is more evident in males, for whom orgasm and morning penile erections decrease progressively from adolescence. By contrast, if anything, older women may enjoy enhanced response when free of the consequence of child-bearing, and due to clitoral enlargement after the menopause. Earlier generations, however, were brought up differently, and may women find it difficult to enjoy sex for its own sake. They relate their feelings much more to childbirth, than do men, so that having children is often satisfaction enough.

The Kinsey report showed that older men whose frequency of orgasm had dropped markedly could reverse this decline with new partners, new techniques, or new sources of outlet, since loss of interest is produced by repetition of the same sort of experience. The dangers of sexual intercourse have often been exaggerated. When questioned, prostitutes who deal with older clients have reported negligible harm to them. While the physiological demands of intercourse can be quite high in the young, with heart rates of 170/min and blood pressures reaching 250/120 mmHg (33/16 kPa), in the long-married older person, the heart rate may only reach 120/min for 10–15 seconds, which is well within his capacity. It follows from this that, following myocardial infarction, some modification or extra-marital experience is wise.

Closeness enhances the personal sense of being valued as a man or woman. The new generation of old people can be expected to view sex positively and will expect informed advice. The advocacy of HRT is part of this higher expectation.

It is not impossible, by any means, to experience sexual satisfaction for the first time in old age, or to have this dimension of living reported. The longer sexual activity has been abandoned, the more difficult it is to restore, but, even where infirmity prevents normal intercourse, other forms of sensual enhancement can provide closeness and the sense of being valued as a man or a woman.

Renewed intercourse in late life may bring medical problems, usually presenting as gynaecological problems. Vaginal discharge or soreness may be a sign of sexual difficulty, and older women are grateful for advice on the use of oestrogen creams and lubricant gels. Among older men, there is a marked discrepancy between the number of morning erections and the ability to have intercourse. Psychological factors are often uppermost here and time should be spent providing reassurance. Testosterone therapy is useless and may be dangerous. Probably less than 5% of men become eunuchoid following castration for prostatic carcinoma, the adrenal cortex continuing to provide sufficient androgen to maintain normal sexual function.

All who deal with these matters should point out that, as age advances, a man may have fewer organisms, but his ability to maintain an erection is usually enhanced, so that he may satisfy female partners better than the young.

Finally, the boarding school attitude to sex raises the suitability of many residential homes when re-housing old people. The separation of married couples and the failure to understand the problems posed for the life-long homosexual individual, derive from outdated mores and impoverished training methods.

ALTERED BOWEL FUNCTION

Most cases of altered bowel habit can be readily diagnosed after a meticulous history and careful examination, followed by sigmoidoscopy and barium enema. The empirical use of drugs is not to be recommended.

Altered bowel habit is frequently seen in elderly patients and is well-known as an indication of serious pathology. In taking the history, one has to be precise about what is meant by terms such as 'diarrhoea' and 'constipation' which have different meanings to different patients. Of particular relevance is the change from one state to the other. Having clarified the frequency and consistency of the motions, enquiry should then pass on to include associated symptoms, such as tenesmus, abdominal pain, blood, etc., and the type of food eaten and its source. Enquiry should include drugs and past medical history, including abdominal operations, such as partial gastrectomy which was quite common in the 1950's. The appearance of the patient may indicate dehydration, cachexia, anaemia or jaundice. Other signs may be helpful, such as spider naevi, acanthosis nigricans and pigmentation of the abdominal flanks, which may indicate pancreatic carcinoma. The field is very wide and will include anxiety, depression and lack of exercise, as well as systemic diseases, such as thyroid disorders, and diabetes mellitus which may have produced autonomic neuropathy, often associated with diarrhoea which usually occurs when the patient lies down. In the elderly, one also has to remember conditions such as ischaemic colitis which is often associated with irregular bowel habits and which usually presents with sudden bouts of loose stools, containing fresh blood or clots, and abdominal pain. It has to be differentiated from diseases such as Crohn's disease, which has a second peak of incidence over the age of 70, as well as acute diverticulitis and proctocolitis. These situations are therefore urgent, particularly diarrhoea, where they may be hypokalaemia and hyponatraemia, and loss of alkaline reserve, so that lethargy and confusion may result, requiring urgent hospital admission to deal with the electrolyte imbalance. It must also be remembered that, in the elderly, constipation may eventually lead to faecal impaction, and, in turn, to spurious diarrhoea, urinary incontinence, and even mental confusion.

Incontinence

This is a common, and yet occult, condition, many believing it to be an inevitable accompaniment of ageing which must be endured, while others are ashamed of having lost control of micturition. The patient may also feel that loss of social capacity may lead to loss of independence which will force him into institutional care. Every attempt should be made to treat the patient in his own home provided that the type and cause of incontinence is known and understood. Relatives and principal helpers are favourably influenced by the demonstration of optimistic and positive planning by members of the primary health care team. Accepting the symptom, reassuring the patient, and defining the type of incontinence are the key to successful management. The GP can ask the patient the following questions:

* Can you remember how long you have had this trouble? (The rate of onset helps identify the precipitating cause of what is usually an acute or chronic condition. A long history suggests a chronic, worsening condition, and the patient now starts to complain at a threshold. Preceding factors, the voiding pattern by day and by night, and specific times are helpful, since nocturia indicates problems of bladder capacity and of fluid retention, as in cardiac failure.)
* Did it come on gradually, or were you affected suddenly?
* Was it connected with any particular event? (A fall, after operation, the menopause, a stroke, a change in a prescribed drug.)
* How much warning do you get?
* Are you drinking more or less than usual?
* Do you feel a need to pass urine more often during the day? How often? How often at night?
* Do you wet yourself without knowing it? If so, is it much?
* Do you have a leakage of urine when you laugh, cough, sneeze, or turn over in bed?
* Do you dribble after passing urine?
* Do you feel you are able to empty the bladder completely?
* Do you have any trouble with your bowels?
* Have you noticed anything unusual about your urine?

A rough estimate of intake and output gives an indication of water load, or the presence of dehydrating illness.

Involuntary micturition suggests a neurological cause, while retention with overflow suggests prostatic hypertrophy, pelvic tumour or faecal impaction.

It is important to notice such psychological factors as shame, indifference, anger or depression in the attitude of the patient, and, indeed, dementia, and the attitudes of relatives, e.g. rejection, acceptance, resignation. Finally, it is worth enquiring about the drug regime for such drugs as diuretics, sedatives, anticholinergics and sympathomimetics.

The home visit

It is important to establish the composition of the home and the patient's place within it. If the first visit of the patient is to the practice centre, a home visit by the practice nurse should be requested. The object of the home visit is to look at the suitability of the home:

> Does the patient have free access to the whole house?
> Is there an odour of urine?
> Is the house tidy, or is there evidence of neglect?
> What happens to soiled linen?
> Does the patient spend all the time in night clothes?
> Is there good lighting, constant hot water, and all round warmth in winter?
> Is he more than 15 paces from the toilet?
> Could the height of the toilet, bed or chair be improved?
> Is he hoarding drugs?
> Is the way to the toilet well lit, safe and obstacle free?
> Or does the patient have to climb stairs?
> Is there a heat source so that cold does not act as a deterrent?
> Is it easy to enter in a hurry?
> Is the door wide enough to allow entry with a walking aid?
> Is the toilet shared with others? If so, by how many?
> Does he indeed know his way to the toilet?
> Does he know where the light switches and handles are?
> Would a sign on the door be helpful?
> *The toilet*
> Does the door open and close easily?
> Could an arthritic patient manage the light switch?
> Or would a cord pull be helpful?
> Is the seat at the right height, and can he raise and lower it?
> Are handrails needed?
> Can the patient operate the flush system?
> Is it advisable to install an alarm or call system for confidence?
> Is the floor covering suitable for easy cleaning?

When to refer

Because the primary condition must be treated, as well as the secondary effects, such as infection, there are many instances when patients need to be referred for further investigation. This may be to a rheumatologist, cardiologist, endocrinologist, neurologist or radiologist. Patients with local lesions should be referred to a urologist, or gynaecologist. The main reason for specialist referral is to obtain a voiding cystometrogram, which is most useful for male patients some months after prostatectomy, and those with unstable tonic and atonic bladder problems. The referral letter should contain the following information:

> How long the patient has had the symptoms,
> Type of onset,
> Fluid intake and urinary output,
> Presumptive diagnosis and the investigations carried out,
> Home conditions, family relationships,
> Premorbid personalities/mental condition,
> Related diseases
> Drug therapy,
> Reason for referral.

Management

Professional help will be needed from the following sources if available:

> Incontinence Nursing Adviser
> The Community Nurse
> The Rehabilitation Nurse
> Voluntary help

The incontinent patient must be treated with the same respect as if his symptoms were a cough or a headache. Wherever possible, he should get up each day and be dressed in day clothes. Fluid should not be restricted and constipation should be avoided. Alcohol, sedatives and hypnotics should be avoided, and, wherever possible, the patient should be relieved of guilt feeling. If he is depressed, appropriate treatment must be offered.

Drug treatment

Many drugs influence detrusor and urethral smooth muscle activity. Unfortunately, the effects of these drug treatments are variable in the elderly, and side-effects may occur.

* Anticholinergic drugs reduce the contractility of the detrusor and are therefore of most value in patients with irritable or unstable bladders.
* α-Adrenergic antagonists may be of help in managing patients with poor voiding ability.
* β-Adrenergic agents may be combined with propantheline for the treatment of unstable bladders.
* Cholinergic drugs may be used in selected patients with neurogenic bladder problems. The atonic detrusor may be made to contract and to produce spontaneous voiding, but caution is urged because this may cause severe side-effects.
* Oestrogens are very effective when used locally in atrophic urethritis and vaginitis. Oral preparations may be used for action on the bladder trigone.
* Antibiotics can be given at intervals in rotation to control odour. Hexamine hippurate is preferred because it avoids the problem of resistant organisms where there is ascending infection.

There are many appliances available, but confused or demented patients often interfere with them. Kanga pants are the best design to keep urine away from the skin.

Catheterization with indwelling catheter is used as a last resort, for instance in unconscious patients, and they require regular irrigation.

Perineal floor exercises, however useful in younger women, are not worth recommending to the elderly, except as placebo.

Where the passage of urine can be anticipated, the patient can be kept dry by regular voiding. The nurse should be asked to chart the amount and type of urine passed.

Follow-up

There are two kinds of incontinent patient, and both types should be followed up.

(1) *Reversible incontinence (D.A.M.P.):*
    Diuresis due to drugs,

Osmotic diuresis caused by hyperglycaemia, hypercalcaemia, and renal failure,
Atrophy, e.g. senile vaginitis,
Mechanical problems,
Psychological problems.
(2) *Irreversible incontinence which may be caused by (P.I.S.S.):*
Prostatectomy,
Inhibition failure, e.g. dementia,
Spinal lesions,
Sensation loss.

ACUTE CONFUSION

Confusion is a descriptive term and not a diagnosis. We should regard it in the same way that we speak of the term 'convulsion' in children.

Confusion indicates disordered awareness of the surroundings and a fluctuating level of consciousness in which erroneous percepts may appear as reality to the patient. Attention is impaired and visual hallucinations and delusions are not uncommon, particularly when poor illumination makes clear stereoscopic vision difficult in identifying objects. Confusion may be interrupted by apparent clear periods, and Brocklehurst has compared the state to being in a fog, seeing only here and there patches of a building, tree or motor car, without being able to relate them to each other.

It is important, therefore, that acute confusion is clearly distinguished from dementia, since one is acute and reversible; the other chronic and irreversible. Of course, patients with dementia are not always confused, even though they are predisposed to be so by functional reserve capacity. Such capacity of most organs is reduced by age, but, while acute confusional states can occur in those previously of normal state (including the young), acute confusion is more likely to be superimposed on those whose mental function is already impaired.

The history, obtained from relatives, friends or neighbours, is therefore important in determining whether one is dealing with an acute state or a chronic and irreversible state of brain failure. Associated features, such as self-neglect and incontinence, urinary or faecal, are helpful in the differentiation. However, it is important to gather details of the past medical history and, in particular, any medication. The clinical examination is of cardinal importance because acute confusional states may complicate a great breadth of pathologies:

Toxic, especially chest infections and alcohol,
Failed homeostasis, e.g. diabetes, hepatic failure, dehydration,
Change of environment,
Faecal impaction,
Severe pain,
Carcinomatosis,
Drug-induced,
Intracerebral causes, e.g. cerebral oedema, TIA, drug abuse,
Suddenly reduced brain nutrition, e.g. cardiovascular, respiratory, blood loss, hypotension, hypoglycaemia.

HYPOTHERMIA

Accidental hypothermia is diagnosed when the core temperature falls to 35°C or below. It may affect anyone exposed to low ambient temperature, immersion in cold water or damp clothing. Those most vulnerable are at the extremes of life. There is evidence that the condition is declining because socioeconomic conditions are improving, and because of increased awareness of the risks and complications.

Even so, many cases are not recognized before hospital admission. Old people become facultative poikilothermics, failing to appreciate conditions of cold and their insidious effects which are accelerated in many instances by clinical disorders that produce vasodilatation, impair mobility, depress metabolism and reduce awareness. The greatest threat oc-

> I was called to a famous hotel in Surrey where a 74-year-old lady was threatened with eviction by the manager because she persisted in the belief that motor cyclists had gathered under her window to make a noise and annoy her. Six doctors had been called, and each had looked out and reported seeing nothing. As the last doctor available in the district, her desperate son asked me to go. I chose not to negate her delusion, but said it must be distressing for her. Following the establishment of a relationship which did not cast me as an agent of the conspiracy, I asked if I could examine her. As I took away the blanket wrapped around her knees, I saw gross bilateral oedema was present in the ankles. Diuretic therapy was introduced, and, 48 hours later, she reported that the motor cyclists had departed the day before.

After two weeks' leave, I was asked to see a 73-year-old man whose family was worried about his failing mind. He had been alright when I left, and had been seen in my absence and given various medications to sedate him. Although he recognized me, he was totally confused. As he mounted the stairs to prepare for my examination, I followed him, and noted Kussmaul-type breathing. Beneath the bed, was a chamber pot full to the brim with urine. A Labstick indicated glycosuria and ketonuria. When visited in hospital, he confided to me that the people in white coats were not really doctors, but actors, masquerading. His diabetes was not controlled, and I suggested he should be discharged. This was agreed and his mind returned to normal in his familiar surroundings. He wrote later to apologise to the staff, in case he had been rude.

A call was received from a 67-year-old patient requesting a visit to her 90-year-old mother who had come to live with them 6 weeks before but who had not yet been registered. The problem was that for the past two days she had risen at 4 a.m. in order to make tea for the family, and she appeared confused. On arrival, I was shown a piece of knitting which the daughter gave her for amusement. It consisted of coloured squares, joined together each day, but, for the past week, deterioration had set in. Taking the history, I learned that they had noticed she was short of breath climbing the stairs, and had found some tablets from her previous doctor labelled 'For the Heart'. They had given her six of these tablets daily. A telephone call to her previous GP confirmed that these were digoxin 0.25 mg. The patient's daughter was asked not to give any more tablets but to start some more knitting. Five days later, the early morning tea making had stopped and the knitting had returned to its former precision.

curs between the small hours of the morning until midmorning. Feeling normally warm skin on the abdomen or axilla to be cold to the touch requires accurate measurement of the core temperature with a low-reading thermometer used *per rectum*, or, occasionally, in urine voided into a container of low heat conductivity.

The full-blown picture, with pale skin, puffy features, slow cerebration and bradyarrhythmia, associated with gruff speech, resembles myxoedema. A falling blood pressure is a grave sign, heralding circulatory failure.

Not only are those with lower body temperatures less capable of reducing heat loss than those with normal body temperatures, but older subjects are less able to respond to a drop in temperature by increasing oxygen consumption and heat production. The ability to shiver is greatly reduced in old age, as is sensitivity to the discomfort of being cold, while the temperature regulating centre in the hypothalamus becomes less sensitive to peripheral input.

Numerous physical, social and mental factors predispose old people to the risk of hypothermia, which is a condition where prevention is better than cure. It is worthwhile, therefore, for the primary care team to develop a policy which will identify those at risk in advance of winter.

A short list of predisposing factors is helpful, but this is by no means inclusive of all the physical factors:

(1) *Social*
    Living alone,
    Poor housing and heating,
    Excessive alcohol intake.
(2) *Mental*
    Depression,
    Confusion,
    Dementia.
(3) *Physical*
    Endocrine, especially diabetes, hypothyroid state
    Neurological: stroke, Parkinson's disease, impaired consciousness, etc.
    Locomotor: conditions affecting mobility and stability,
    Chronic debilitating conditions, e.g. malignancy, infections,
    Cardiovascular: MI, hyperdynamic circulation, CCF, etc.,
    Respiratory: reduced respiratory reserve capacity,
    Renal and urinary: urinary incontinence, polyuria,

GI tract: chronic diarrhoea, malabsorption, subnutrition,
Drugs: those affecting consciousness.

Prognosis

This depends on body core temperature, so that the mortality rises from about 1/3 of cases between 33°C and 35°C, to 3/4 of those with a body temperature below 30°C.

The Department of Health recommends a standard room temperature of 21.1°C for elderly people, which is rarely met, but the minimum safe temperature is 18.3°C. It requires more heat to maintain warm rooms at the tops of buildings than on the lower floors. Old people and their relatives need instruction in maintaining body warmth by wearing insulated light clothing and a hat indoors and in bed, while avoiding heat loss by confounding the myth that alcohol 'keeps out the cold'. Regular hot drinks, food taken several times a day, and the use of an electric overblanket is effective and economical.

Severe cases of hypothermia require management in the intensive care unit. Mild cases, with a core temperature near 35°C, can be managed at home by giving warm drinks, providing warm blanket insulation, and encouraging mobility.

HYPERTHERMIA

Hyperthermia is not often encountered in the UK. Impaired regulatory function with an increase in the threshold for sweating is the basis for the adverse effects of high environmental temperatures on the elderly population. However, in this country, a sustained hot spell, 26°C, will begin first to produce cases of ischaemic heart disease deaths in 48 hours, and cerebrovascular accidents after a week. This was the case in Athens during the summer of 1987. During weeks of exceptionally hot weather in the southern United States during the summer of 1980, there was a high mortality from heat stroke in old people, with rectal temperatures measuring over 40°C, signs of dehydration, coma, and pulmonary infection.

References

Langford, HG and Watson, RL. (1982). Obesity and hypertension. In Sleight, P and Freis, E. (eds) *Cardiology-Hypertension*. pp. 340–346 (Butterworths)

Sleight, P. (1983). Hypertension. In Wetherall, DJ, Ledingham, GG and Warrell, DA. (eds) *Oxford Textbook of Medicine*, Vol.13, pp. 258–260 (Oxford)

Thompson, MK. (1983). Incontinence in the elderly. In *Medicine in Practice*, pp. 773–777

Thompson, MK. (1983). Decision in Geriatrics. Modern Medicine (October 1983–January 1985)

Section 4
Specialty Aspects

CARDIOVASCULAR DISEASE

Cardiovascular disease in the elderly creates enormous health care needs. Of all the elderly people in the population, more than half suffer from some form of it. About 60% of deaths in persons over 65 are attributable to it and case fatality rates increase with age. The majority of elderly patients admitted to hospital suffer from cardiovascular disease, either as the main or as a corollary reason for admission. Hypertension continues as a powerful risk factor into old age, and elevated lipid levels remain as risk factors for the elderly, although to a lesser extent than in the young and middle-aged.

Normal ageing of the cardiovascular system follows programmed and random patterns affecting the contractile and distensile properties of the myocardium. Pacemaker cells and beta-adrenergic receptors decrease in number and function. Atheromatosis increases with age, with thickening and fibrosis stiffening the arterial tree. Cardiac output is reduced due to lower stroke volume and heart rate caused by autonomic system changes, increasing vascular resistance and decreasing myocardial compliance.

While cardiovascular disease cannot be prevented, it can be delayed in time and intensity by measures which should obviously have started earlier in life:

* Body weight should be kept as close to normal as possible.
* A balanced diet with reduced amount of fat is essential.
* Salt intake should not exceed 5 g daily.
* Smoking should be discouraged, but, if abandonment creates stress, it is doubtful if the benefit outweighs the harm.
* Appropriate exercise within prescribed limits should be encouraged.

A diagnosis of heart disease at any age is an alarming and disturbing event, but it is not unusual for the elderly patient to be treated with less consideration than younger people because a favourable outcome seems to be of less importance. Terms such as 'heart failure' are more threatening to the patient than in the mind of the physician. The confidence of patients who have attacks of arrhythmia, or Stokes Adams attacks may be so undermined that they will not venture out any more. In elderly people, emphasis should be placed on rehabilitation rather than on treatment, and this should be phased in relation to immediate and short-term goals, rather than distant and immediately unattainable ones. Confidence that medical care will be readily available whenever and wherever the patient needs it should not be carried to the point where excessive dependency on the GP or hospital is encouraged.

Admission to hospital for a short period for close observation may be more effective than a longer period as an outpatient. Home care remains the best means of looking after the elderly cardiovascular patient and should be encouraged. The success of drug treatment, which involves compliance, is most at risk when the patient is cared for at home. Simplification, rationalization, and regular clinical review of the treatment are essential. If certain precautions are taken, an elderly person with cardiovascular disease can be allowed to travel provided a certain length of time since the acute stage of the disease has produced equilibrium.

Cardiac surgery may be of great benefit in well-selected patients, no matter how old they may be. But, if a patient is to undergo surgery for another condition, careful assessment and preparation are required before the operation, and considerable care afterwards.

The usual causes of chronic heart failure in the elderly are ischaemic or hypertensive; less often, aortic or other valve disease, or a metabolic or infective disturbance. Anginal pain in the elderly is more difficult to differentiate from other diagnoses than in the younger patient, but the drugs used are the same, although side-effects occur more frequently in the elderly, e.g. orthostatic hypotension and increased intraocular pressure.

In myocardial infarction, chest pain is frequently absent, so that the leading signs may not be the same as in younger patients. Arrhythmia, mental confusion, acute cardiac failure, pulmonary congestion and oedema are the most common early complications in patients over 70 years of age. The fatality rate increases with age. Nevertheless, rehabilitation should commence early. Those susceptible to deconditioning as a result of inactivity are in special need of rehabilitative measures, and psychological care, education and counselling are important components of a rehabilitation programme. The best programme is progressive walking, but exercise training takes longer to produce an effect in the elderly. Hot and humid environments should be avoided, and exercise is encouraged within the limits of tiredness, shortness of breath and chest pain.

Patients over 75 with stable angina respond well to medication and should remain on treatment. Surgery may be considered after judging how active the patient is and how likely this will continue after recovery from surgery. Severe or unstable angina, or critical lesions revealed by coronary cineangiography in patients with fewer symptoms, reinforce the indication for surgery.

The main forms of arrhythmia are sick sinus syndrome, atrial fibrillation, and conduction defects, which occur with greater frequency in the elderly. Some arrhythmias result from age changes but others are caused by various associated diseases. The prognosis for symptomatic arrhythmias is poor, and antiarrhythmic therapy is complicated by the fact that the drugs prescribed, e.g. digitalis, may themselves cause arrhythmias. There is no age limit to the implantation of a pacemaker, the guiding principles being the same as for younger patients.

Valvular disease is common in the elderly due to underlying conditions, such as rheumatic heart disease, syphilis, calcification, mucoid degeneration, and papillary muscle dysfunction. Aortic valve diseases, incompetence and stenosis are the most frequently encountered. If they occur as a consequence of ageing, they carry a good prognosis. Surgical correction may be considered, even for older patients, if symptoms curtail the activities of daily living.

The bizarre and confusing clinical picture produced by infective endocarditis must not be overlooked because the prognosis is poor, and the consequences so serious prophylactic measure should be instituted whether or not the patient is considered to be at risk. The incidence is increasing in the elderly, and the treatment is similar to that for younger patients.

The heart is involved in chronic lung disease, and persistent elevation of pulmonary artery pressure results in chronic cor pulmonale. Cigarette smoking is the principal contributing factor, and means of prevention and treatment include avoiding exposure to indoor pollution and indoor crowds, early treatment of infection with antibiotics, relieving bronchospasm, oxygen therapy, and treating heart failure. Such patients should be singled out especially for vaccination against influenza before an impending epidemic. Finally, respiratory depressants, e.g. morphine, should never be prescribed for patients with obstructive lung disease, particularly the elderly.

Diseases of the veins

Varicose veins are common and treatment is mainly conservative. Surgery and sclerotherapy are rarely recommended over the age of 60.

Phlebitis is treated with elastic bandaging and non-steroidal anti-inflammatory drugs. DVT occurs frequently after surgery or after hip fracture, and may result in a potentially fatal pulmonary embolism.

Pulmonary embolism

Pulmonary embolism, when suspected, should be treated by 10,000 iu heparin by intravenous infusion without delay, unless a major contraindication is present. In the elderly, it is often difficult to distinguish between pulmonary embolism and pneumonia, but correct timely diagnosis and treatment can be life saving, not only as an immediate measure, but in preventing further embolization. Minor pulmonary embolism may become manifest as transitory dyspnoea, irregular fever, or as an exacerbation of congestive heart failure. It must be thought of along with thyrotoxicosis when fast atrial fibrillation resists attempts to control it with digoxin.

Anticoagulants

Anticoagulant therapy is used with caution in elderly patients because of frequent haemorrhagic complications. It may be continued for the patient's life in such conditions as arterial embolism where a cardiac source persists, and in mitral stenosis, although it may be discontinued after valvotomy.

Peripheral arterial disease

The patient is usually male and over 40. Almost all are smokers, and one third have already had a myocardial infarction by the time they present with peripheral arterial disease. Almost all eventually die from coronary heart disease, one third are hypertensive, and 10% are diabetic. The patient should be encouraged to 'walk through' his claudication pain. Vasodilator drugs are disappointing, but a graduated exercise programme tends to increase walking distance provided smoking is abandoned. Few, in fact, require surgical intervention.

CEREBROVASCULAR DISEASE

Stroke mortality rates increase with age in geometrical progression. It affects males and females alike, and, unlike coronary heart disease, affects social classes equally. Mortality rates are conspicuously lower where attention is paid to control of hypertension and diabetes. Aspirin, given in low doses, and platelet anti-aggregants may be useful in high-risk patients, especially following a transient ischaemic attack. When a patient has extracranial artery disease, e.g. carotid artery stenosis, surgery can prevent stroke.

When the patient is unconscious, a number of other conditions should be considered. Death usually occurs in four days where unconsciousness is prolonged. When the patient is conscious, the clinical diagnosis of stroke as such is reliable, but the type of stroke is often difficult to diagnose.

Except in mild or very severe cases, the patient should be referred to hospital as an emergency case with full information of past medical history and current medication. Special stroke units have a greater success in treating and rehabilitating patients than the general medical ward.

Barriers to recovery are particularly present in strokes affecting the less dominant hemisphere, when the first thing to establish is whether spacial perception has been disturbed. Other barriers are motor and sensory disturbances, impaired communication, balance disturbance, depression, and, very often, interference with intellectual function and emotional incontinence.

RESPIRATORY DISEASE

Between 50 and 70 years, cardiorespiratory efficiency is markedly reduced due to chest wall rigidity, a decrease in arterial oxygen tension, and a great increase in residual volume.

Chronic bronchitis and pulmonary emphysema do exist separately, but are often related. The great thing here is to prevent acute on chronic infection by urging patients to stop smoking, and offering influenza vaccine prophylactically. Patients can be trained to recognize the significance of increased sputum production and can be given antibiotics to keep in order to start a course early when needed.

Treatment of bronchospasm is important, but theophylline drugs, recently enjoying renewed popularity, are again under a cloud as they are suspected of being toxic. Absorption is also very variable so that the correct dose is difficult to calculate. Pressurized nebulizers are difficult for old people to use, but a nebuhaler and a β_2-stimulating drug is easier.

Bronchial asthma, although less common in the elderly, can occur for the first time, and treatment is the same as in the young.

Pneumonia

Pneumonia remains a formidable problem for primary care physicians who either treat it or may feel that treatment is best omitted in certain conditions, such as dementing illness, where medical wisdom is often preferable to medical knowledge. Factors contributing to the severity of pneumonia in aged patients are:

- The virulence of the respiratory pathogen,
- The host's defensive capability,
- The speed of application of medical treatment,
- The patient's pulmonary reserve,
- The presence of concomitant disease and its severity.

Predisposition occurs in patients with the following chronic conditions:

- Chronic obstructive airways disease (COAD),
- Pulmonary neoplasm,
- Chronic alcoholism,
- Chronic congestive cardiac failure,
- Recent influenzal infection,
- Swallowing disorders,
- Immunoglobulin deficiencies.

Aged patients with pneumonia are apt to be afebrile, even when there is bacteraemia. The anticipated 'classical' physical signs do not invariably present in elderly patients, but a respiratory rate over 24/minute has been significantly associated with pneumonia. Such aspects as pleuritic pain, productive cough, dyspnoea, lethargy, etc. may be masked by changes in the patient's mental status. Pneumonia can also be accompanied by exacerbation of coexistent diseases, such as coronary heart disease, chronic congestive heart failure or chronic obstructive lung disease.

Diagnosis, therefore, depends heavily upon the chest X-ray. However, good films are often difficult to obtain in elderly patients who are confused, agitated or severely dyspnoeic. Radiologically, pneumonia can stimulate congestive cardiac failure, pulmonary embolism, and the adult respiratory distress syndrome in the aged.

Other things to bear in mind in the differential diagnosis are neoplasia, pneumonitis (caused by radiation), hypersensitivity, and drugs. The situation may be clarified by serial X-rays, inhalation–perfusion scan and fibre-optic bronchoscopy. A complete blood count is often of limited diagnostic value, but blood cultures should be obtained prior to the onset of therapy in both febrile and afebrile patients.

Bacteriology

The leading cause of pneumonia in the community is *Streptococcus pneumoniae*, and the second most common cause in patients living at home is *Haemophilus influenzae*. Other recognized bacterial causes include *Legionella*, *Staphylococcus aureus*, Group-B *streptococci*, *Klebsiellae*, and *Baranhamella catarrhalis*, formerly known as *Neisseria catarrhalis*. For these reasons, it is important to obtain a sputum for culture to identify the aetiological agent in case there is failure to respond to the first antimicrobial treatment offered. However, this is often difficult in frail elderly patients with a poor cough reflex.

Supportive measures

It is not always necessary to keep the patients in bed. They may be sat high enough for them to stand occasionally and even walk a few steps. Attention should be paid to the possibility of protein-calorie malnutrition and particularly to dehydration. There is also the obligation to attend to coexistent problems, such as arrhythmias, angina, diabetes, and even empyema, while adjusting the dose of any immunosuppressive drug being taken in order to maximize the patient's own defences. It is unwise to prescribe antipyretic agents and care must be taken in the use of cough medicines and narcotics because of their tendency to suppress the cough reflex as well as the respiratory drive. Needless to say, all elderly people should receive polyvalent influenza vaccine annually. But data suggests that the elderly often fail to develop protective antibody from the pneumococcal vaccine, which has not proved efficacious.

The role of physiotherapy remains debatable, but there is little doubt of the value of postural drainage in patients not too weak to undertake it, particularly after the administration of oxygen, which has been shown to impair muco-ciliary transport and to cause pulmonary fibrosis.

Table 4.1 Antibiotic therapy

Organism	Primary therapy	Alternative therapy	Duration of therapy
Strep. pneumoniae	Mild: oral penicillin V Mod. to severe: IM procaine penicillin G	Erythromycin, oral or IV	1 week
Haem. influenzae	Ampicillin	Cephalosporin or chloramphenicol	2 weeks
Gram –ve aerobic bacilli	Amyloglycoside + 3rd generation cephalsporin or semi-synthetic pencillin	IV Trimethoprim-sulphamethazole	2–3 weeks
Staph. aureus	Methicillin	Vanocomycin or trimethoprim-sulphamethoxazole	2–3 weeks
Legionella pneumophila	IV Erythromycin	IV Doxycycline + rifampicin in severe illness	3 weeks
Anaerobes	IV Penicillin	IC Clindamycin	10 days
Branhamella catarrhalis	IV Erythromycin	IV Doxycycline	10 days

Footnote: Note that in the patient who has a significant reaction to penicillin, it is prudent to avoid the cephalosporins; for such patients, erythromycin is the drug of choice.

DISORDERS OF THE ALIMENTARY SYSTEM

False teeth need to be well maintained and occasionally replaced due to changes in the shape of the mandible with age. Some geriatricians relate poor nutrition to the edentulous state, but, having found patients who only wear then when I visit and are well nourished, I cannot believe this to be true. More important considerations are the cosmetic effects. Dental hygiene is important in avoiding suppurative parotitis.

The oesophagus

About 60% of old people have a hiatus hernia but pain occurs only when there is oesophagitis. Most respond to a regime of postural and dietary advice and simple antacids. If not, H_2-antagonists can be used. One of the most common complications of oesophagitis is a benign stricture requiring bougeinage at regular intervals.

Peptic ulcer

Duodenal ulcers (DUs) reach a peak prevalence in middle age in men, falling off later, perhaps due to declining gastric acid production. In women, this decline does not occur, so that the prevalence of gastric ulcers (GUs) becomes similar to that of DUs. The presentation may be iron deficiency anaemia or non-specific weight loss, rather than the typical dyspeptic symptomatology. For DUs, the H_2 antagonists are the treatment of choice, but, for GUs, tri-potassium dicitrato bismuthate (De-nol) is preferred. Carbenoxolone, with its salt and water retentive properties and lowering of potassium, should not be used.

Gallstones

Surgery should not be sought in patients who have no symptoms. It should only be considered for those with previous episodes of acute cholecystitis. Occasionally, medical treatment with ursodeoxycholic acid is recommended, but only 40% of gall stones are suitable, and, since in old people there is a high recurrence rate, once started, the treatment should continue.

Jaundice

Drug toxicity ranks about equal with cancer of the biliary tract as a leading cause of cholestatic jaundice, and the condition responds when the offending drug, of which there is a wide range, is stopped.

Malabsorption sometimes develops for the first time in old age as a late complication of previous gastric surgery, but it may occur in a number of other conditions, such as chronic inflammatory and malignant disorders, small bowel diverticulae, chronic pancreatitis, and coeliac disease.

Diverticular disease

Diverticular disease of the colon is the most common disorder of the large bowel, but it is important to make sure that symptoms and X-ray appearances are linked before embarking upon a long course of treatment.

Less common conditions, such as ulcerative colitis, Crohn's disease and ischaemic colitis, must all be considered in older people.

Laxative abuse

The only way to find out about the reality of this is to enquire at the local pharmacy. I have found that the sale of laxatives over the counter has fallen greatly since the attachment of health visitors and dieticians able to provide the patients with rational advice.

Faecal incontinence

This is most commonly due to faecal impaction or diarrhoea. Very rare cases require surgery for rectal prolapse or lax sphincter. Its association with dementia is rare in the community, but may be well controlled by the use of codeine phosphate and clearing the colon once a week with a phosphate enema.

THE LOCOMOTOR SYSTEM

Joint disorders

Rheumatoid arthritis can be of long standing, when pain and disability may be due more to joint deformity than active disease. In about 10% of cases, the disease begins for the first time in patients of 60 and over. In the majority of these, the signs and symptoms are classical, but a quarter of them present as the 'benign rheumatoid arthritis of the aged' which has an excellent prognosis with remission after 18 months, despite a severe onset.

Drug treatment is the same as in the young where there is involvement of the synovia, but attention must be paid to increased toxicity, interactions with other preparations, and compliance. It is ironic that the greater the anti-inflammatory effect, the greater the risk of mucosal erosion and ulceration. Perhaps those drugs with long half-lives, such as fenbufen and naproxen, have some advantage in the elderly.

While gout affects males predominantly in early middle age, the sexes approach equality of incidence in late life. The management of an acute exacerbation is the same for the old as for the young. Uricosuric agents are not advocated for long-term treatment of patients with reduced life expectancy. There is, in any case, a tendency for serum uric acid levels to be higher, particularly for those on diuretics.

Osteoarthritis is very common. There is little correlation between radiological signs and patient symptoms. The dilemma in treatment is whether effective drug treatment, including intra-articular hydrocortisone, allows too much use to be made of a joint. There are those who work through their pain until it is lost, so that each case must be judged individually. Pain is rarely constant, and drugs, therefore, can be given intermittently. Passive movement of the joints and exercises, such as straight leg raising, are important to maintain muscular integrity, which, once lost, is almost impossible to regain. It is worth doing the ESR when joints are severely inflamed, and it should be noted that prolonged immobility in a fixed flexed position often causes more pain than overuse of a joint – another argument for the rocking chair! Having never seen exercise produce a Charcot type of joint, and considering the morale-raising effect of exercise, exercise is to be encouraged – particularly in women after a warm bath.

Bone disorders

Osteoporosis favours thin North European women who smoke. Its prevention begins in early life, encouraging a good bone mass, with HRT following the menopause. Since obesity seems to be a preventive, apart from delayed fall in oestrogens, gravitational factors must play a part. Therefore, older women should be instructed to keep active, avoid resting unduly, and maintain an adequate calcium intake of 1 g daily. The danger is liability to fracture, not only of the arm and hip, but crush fractures of the vertebrae, most commonly where kyphosis creates undue force on the lower thoracic vertebrae. This is an indication for increased calcium and perhaps a short course of anabolic steroid.

In a country where the angle of the sun from October to April is insufficient to produce Vitamin D, cases of osteomalacia occur, with bone pain, muscle weakness, low calcium and phosphate, but high serum alkaline phosphatase concentrations. Looser's zones on X-ray are diagnostic. There is, perhaps, a case for giving a multivitamin preparation prophylactically to all patients who are housebound. Treatment of osteomalacia is by a single intramuscular injection of 600,000 units of calciferol and calcium supplements if serum calcium is low.

Paget's disease is common in the weight-bearing joints and often found incidentally in radiographs. The complications of deformity leading to deafness, cord compression and fracture are now preventable, but careful assessment is needed to ensure one is not treating heart failure from other causes, or simply presbyacusis. New methods of treatment with calcitonin and diphosphonate, which are expensive, are best carried out by specialists.

Muscle disorders

Polymyalgia rheumatica involves the muscles of the shoulder and pelvic girdle, and is closely associated with cranial arteritis. It is, therefore, a medical emergency and requires immediate treatment with 45–60 mg prednisolone. It is more common in women, and the striking feature is the periodicity of the symptoms which are maximal early in the morning, after which the pain reduces. The initial high dose can be reduced during the first week to a maintenance dose of 2.5–10 mg daily. The ESR is monitored in order to achieve this, and again a month after cessation of therapy. Normally, one needs to continue for 1 year or 18 months before there is remission.

ENDOCRINE DISORDERS

Thyroid disease

Thyrotoxicosis used to be considered a disease of young women, but 40% of cases are in patients over 60. Misdiagnosis occurs due to atypical presentation, with symptoms that are often vague, such as anorexia, weight loss and associated lassitude – in fact a 'failure to thrive' syndrome, which may be thought natural in an old person. Half these elderly thyrotoxic patients show atrial fibrillation. The most commonly used treatment is radio iodine in larger doses than for the young to ensure relief of cardiac overstimulation. The resulting hypothyroidism is easily supplemented.

Hypothyroidism is a diagnosis often missed in plump elderly women, and 2% of routine hospital admissions have been found to be hypothyroid. Testing for thyroid autoantibodies is a worthwhile procedure in post-menopausal women complaining of weight problems while dieting ineffectively. The treatment of hypothyroidism is essentially the

> The FPC telephoned to ask if we would take on a 78-year-old lady who had been put off the list of a neighbouring colleague. Before we agreed, we asked his reason on the telephone. He stated that he had visited her before morning surgery and received no answer. Being a conscientious man, he had called again at 4 p.m. to find the patient up and dressed, with nothing at all the matter with her. Being a busy man, he could not be bothered with such people.
>
> Next day, a visit was made to the patient who was very anxious not to upset me. She said she had been pinned to her bed by pain when she heard the doctor come the first time, and that he was very angry on the second visit. She had not called any doctor out for 25 years. She went to fill the kettle for a cup of tea at a tap high on the wall. Noticing she poured water over the outside, I helped her and she said she was not seeing too well out of one eye. An injection of 100 mg prednisolone was immediately given, and a follow-up visit next day showed a remarkable improvement. This can sometimes be used as a therapeutic test.

same as for the young except that it is begun with lower doses of thyroxine with slower increases. All the patients treated with ^{131}I for thyrotoxicosis should have thyroid function tests at regular intervals. Only T4 with a raised TSH should be sought as T3 levels are frequently in the normal range, perhaps reflecting a compensatory mechanism. Low T4 levels due to altered protein binding can be recognized by direct estimation of TBG.

Diabetes mellitus

This affects 17% of those over 65 and 26% of those over 85 and its prevalence amongst older people is rising. Glucose tolerance decreases with age, and half those over 70 would have an abnormal blood glucose 2 h after a glucose load. Diagnosis, therefore, depends either on finding elevated fasting glucose levels or symptoms of diabetes, e.g. fungal infection, with a borderline level. A GTT test is needed for confirmation. In practice, diabetes is found in three ways:

(1) As a random finding.
(2) When complications are found.
(3) The disease may present as in the young with weight loss, polydypsia and polyuria, and ketosis.

The insidious onset is dangerous as severe hyperglycaemia may cause dehydration and hyperosmolar non-ketotic coma as the first manifestation. It is advisable to screen all patients more than 20% above ideal body weight, and those with evidence of coronary, cerebral or peripheral vascular disease, cataract or fungal skin infection.

Treatment in most cases is based on diet alone, but, according to the severity of the condition, may be based on diet and oral hypoglycaemic drugs, or diet and insulin therapy. The latter may become necessary during episodes of intercurrent infectious illness, such as pneumonia.

Vascular and neuropathic complications are aggravated by poor control. All older diabetic patients should have proper foot care and be seen periodically by a chiropodist.

Patients should be instructed in methods of testing. Too often, they test urine in the morning when glucose is absent after fasting all night. They should test preferably at night, when a small amount of sugar is a reassurance against hypoglycaemia in the night. Drugs used as oral hypoglycaemic agents are:

(1) Sulphonylureas. These are effective when residual pancreatic b-cells are active. Adverse reactions are common and some are absorbed irregularly. These drugs should be studied carefully.
(2) Biguanides. Metformin, the only such drug now used, is absorbed completely. It is used alone or with a sulphonylurea in those obese patients who cannot be controlled on diet alone. Toxicity is increased where clearance of the drug is delayed, e.g. in renal failure, respiratory insufficiency or liver disease.

Obesity

Nothing, perhaps, causes more frustration between doctor and patient than attempts to manage obesity. Effective weight loss is sometimes only achieved if caloric intake is reduced to 600/day, which makes patients ill. More important is to encourage exercise to increase metabolic rate, but this is also very difficult. Nevertheless, patients should be discouraged from attending clinics where appetite suppressants form part of the management. Occasionally, temporary relief is obtained by going to groups, but many older people in town now fear to go out after dark.

The doctor will, therefore, lose nothing by explaining that the causes of obesity are obscure and protecting the patient against feelings of guilt and ugliness. He will need to explain that good results may take months or years to achieve, and will involve a new style of life. Counselling will help the patient to balance the advantages and disadvantages of such changes. It is a field widely exploited by writers in womens' magazines, and patients should be protected against the claims constantly being made by increasingly bogus diets in a field where it seems that anyone can claim to be an 'expert'. Relief of depression, for which the reward of food of often self-administered, is important, and patients should be handled with delicacy and sensitivity.

THE BLOOD

The blood constituents are not altered by age, except that albumin falls and globulins rise, which may affect ESR values. An ESR up to 45 mm/h is common in both sexes, but tests should be repeated since changes are more important than absolute values.

Anaemia

There is no such thing as a 'physiological' anaemia. Haemoglobin of less than 12.0 g/dl in an elderly person must be considered significant and the prevalence of anaemia does increase with age, more in women than in men.

Iron deficiency anaemia

Iron deficiency anaemia accounts for 45% of elderly anaemic patients and is most likely to be due to blood loss in the GI tract, of which there are many causes ranging from hiatus hernia to haemorrhoids. The first investigation is stool testing for occult blood, repeated perhaps more than once, before other investigations are ordered. The importance of malnutrition as a cause of iron deficiency anaemia has probably been overemphasized in the elderly. On the other hand, minor degrees of malabsorption may occur and the incidence of achlorhydria increases with age. There are also the anaemias associated with diseases, such as rheumatoid disease and malignant disease, to be considered. When iron deficiency has been established and is treated the Hb should return to normal in 6–8 weeks, but treatment should continue for another 3 months to replenish iron stores. In perhaps one third of old people with anaemia, the serum iron concentration is normal. Overt iron deficiency is indicated by SI of less than 60 μg/dl and TIBC higher than 400 μg/dl.

Megaloblastic anaemia

The usual causes of B_{12} deficiency are pernicious anaemia, gastrectomy, and malabsorption due to coeliac disease, but any disease that affects the terminal ileum may be responsible. The association between B_{12} deficiency and mental change is well known, and, in some cases, there is improvement in mental state with B_{12} therapy.

In general practice, the finding of a serum B_{12} level below 1.3 ng/dl is diagnostic of pernicious anaemia and examination of the peripheral blood will show low Hb and an MCV of more than 100 cu/μm. A blood smear reveals macrocytic ovalocytes with marked variation in the size and shape of the red cells. Intrinsic factor antibodies occur in the serum of 60% of patients and are important diagnostically. There is no case for using cyanocobalamin as a 'tonic' for run-down old people except where a deficiency is proven, although daily injections for 1 week seem to reduce the intensity of herpes zoster. Potassium supplements are required in the early treatment of pernicious anaemia because of the formation of new cells in the marrow.

Myeloproliferative disorders are more common in the elderly, the commonest of these disorders being chronic lymphocytic anaemia which may be discovered in a routine blood film for an unrelated disorder, although some patients will have lymph node enlargement and splenomegaly. The appearance of a leuko-erythroblastic picture in the peripheral blood is an indication of metastatic cancer, of which the commonest cause in men is Ca prostate, and in women, Ca breast. Aplastic anaemia is less common in the old than the young, when it occurs, but requires a review of drug therapy.

The plasma cell dyscrasias (monoclonal gammopathies) are increasingly prevalent in the elderly. They include Waldenström's macroglobinaemia, amyloidosis, heavy- and light-chain disease, and the commonest – multiple myeloma, the presenting symptom of which is back pain associated with anaemia. The ESR is almost always more than 100 mm/h.

NEUROLOGICAL DISORDERS

Parkinson's disease

The diagnosis depends upon recognizing two or more of the following signs: tremor, akinesia, rigidity and postural abnormality. It is an important source of disability, such as falling and immobility. Diagnostic difficulties arise because older patients are more heterogeneous, and more likely to develop confusion, incontinence and hypotension with levodopa. Drugs should be reviewed to exclude secondary parkinsonism.

The GP will be more effective if he visits the home and counsels relatives. Drugs and their side effects need careful explanation, and advice is often sought on continuing at work and driving a car. A team assessment of the home will lead to useful suggestions and alterations. Physical management and speech therapy are important adjuncts to drug therapy, the duration of which is limited, for eventually dopaminergic cells degenerate because of pigment overload.

Symptoms do not remain constant and patients will often be entrusted with dose modification to suit their activities, e.g. an extra dose may be taken by a lady arranging for a meeting of friends in her house to avoid becoming over-tired.

It is best to refer all patients to a neurological consultant, for management becomes difficult in the decompensated phase. Much is to be gained by introducing the patient to a local branch of the Parkinson's Disease Society (Head Office, 36 Portland Place, London, W1N 3DG).

Herpes zoster and post-herpetic neuralgia

This is found predominantly in the elderly, and the majority of cases are ophthalmic and geniculate herpes. Post-herpetic pain can be expected over the age of 70. Where the ophthalmic division is involved, the integrity of the cornea is threatened if warning lesions appear along the nasociliary branch, requiring referral unless one is experienced in this condition which may require corticosteroid applications. Herpes-specific enzyme inhibitors, such as acyclovir, are now available for systemic treatment during the first week, and topical agents applied early, such as idoxuridine during the first four days, may shorten the course and prevent or reduce the intensity of post-herpetic symptoms.

The GP will not overlook the probability that herpes zoster may reflect a general lowering of patient immunity, not only to the varicella virus. There is a strong association with chronic leukaemia and the reticuloses.

The disruption of a patient's life by herpetic neuralgia must not be minimized. It may continue for years, either being very acute and intermittent, or felt as unremitting causalgia. All kinds of treatment may be tired, such as vibrators, acupuncture, anti-epileptic and antidepressant drugs, but referral to a pain clinic may have to be made eventually. It is a neurological, not a skin disease.

Degenerative neurological disorders

These are occasionally encountered by all practitioners. Diabetic neuropathy is a difficult problem for which tightening of control is the major therapy.

Alcoholic neuropathy must be born in mind, for it it uncommon, although cases of Korsakoff's psychosis with its dense consistent amnesia occur and may be reversible.

Trigeminal neuralgia is a condition of old age, occurring most commonly in women, and usually responds well to carbamazepine 100 mg daily, which may be increased to 200–300 mg a day if early response is poor.

Motor neurone disease is more common in men and is rarely encountered. It begins with weakness of the hands and shoulders, and, occasionally, speech change. Fasciculation is pathognomonic. A rapid course of two years may produce bulbar symptoms without intellectual deterioration, or the course may be longer and slower.

Neurological changes may be seen in cases of B_{12} deficiency (subacute combined degeneration), Paget's disease and cervical spondylosis. Carcinomatous neuropathy must be considered in cases of obscure aetiology.

MENTAL DISORDERS

Affective disorders

The commonest psychiatric conditions encountered in elderly people are affective disorders. Only in the very aged are organic brain syn-

> An 83-year-old spinster gave up her membership of the bowls club in the middle of the summer. She gave old age as the reason. It was pointed out to her that old age does not strike suddenly. She then volunteered that she was praying at night for forgiveness and could not sleep, for she felt she had to make peace with her Maker before she died. The story emerged that she had once formed an attachment to one young man, and decided she should take him home to introduce him to her stern Victorian father. The young man felt nervous and asked if he could smoke. 'If you do, sir, you will be the first one ever to have done so in this house!' said the father threateningly. The young man left in haste, my patient never forgave her father, and she never married. Now, she felt she had to make amends. Having told her story, she felt relieved, her depression lifted and she returned to the bowls club with renewed energy.

dromes more prevalent. In the aetiology, one is increasingly made to realise that it is the joint combination of biological and psychosocial factors that is important. However, affective disorders are eminently treatable in the old as in the young, but doctors remain less optimistic, and are perhaps less likely to seek therapeutic intervention.

This case suggests that the term endogenous is misleading. Depression is depression at any age and those illnesses which begin in late life are not clearly distinguished from those whose first onset occurs in their younger days. It appears that, while depressive symptoms may be somewhat more common in later life, the prevalence of discrete affective illnesses at this time is probably less than that in earlier life. Knowing when and when not to prescribe is an important art gained by extensive clinical experience of how much present malfunction may be due to present and continuing environmental stress. These skills are insufficiently developed where they can only be acquired, i.e. in general practice.

It seems possible that some changes occur with ageing which may predispose some individuals to depressive illness, such as reduced serotonin activity, although there is no doubt that there is a complex interaction of neurotransmitter systems which may be reflected in different clinical subtypes of depressive illness. The association between hypercortisaemia and depression is well known and the abnormal dexamethasone suppression test (DST) is age related.

Vulnerability to depression is increased in those with physical health problems, and there is increased vulnerability to recent stresses in the socially depressive, which may relate to life-long personality traits and lack of self-esteem. There is an inverse relationship between social class and the prevalence of depressive disorders at all ages, and there is a very wide variation in physical health status between the top and bottom ends of the social stratum. Nevertheless, although social disadvantage and unhappiness may feature together, it is crucial that they are evaluated and treated separately.

Common emotional problems in the elderly

(1) Bereavement and widowhood. By the age of 75, 70% of women are widows. To a fair proportion, after a decent period of 'mourning', widows appear, after the insurance has been paid, wearing new hats and clothes as if a great burden has been lifted from their shoulders! Men hardly ever readapt to the single state. In both sexes, in the immediate bereavement period, the family clusters around, but, after the funeral, friction with family members can arise. Widows often take a relatively long time to grieve for the husbands, and, indeed, may begin to glorify someone who was little more than a cipher. The widow has to renegotiate her relationship with children in a way that places an extra demand on their affection.

(2) Marital problems. The elderly belong to a generation to whom divorce was difficult and where it was thought better to stick it out for the sake of the children, who were not planned in the days before oral contraception. Economic dependence on men also made divorce difficult. Long-standing marital conflict, tolerable when the husband was out at work, is aggravated when retirement takes place and made dramatically worse when mental or physical disability suddenly makes one partner dependent on the other.

(3) Conflicts with children. One frequently hears old women complain about their children's failure to care for them. It is unwise to intervene having heard only one side of the case. When it has been heard, it usually transpires that the neglected parent never fulfilled the role of parent in the first instance.

Long-standing interpersonal difficulties between parents and children are often shelved when the child marries and moves away, but are reactivated when the old parent is bereaved or suffers failty and needs help. This is more than likely when the old person moves into a daughter's or son's home, causing the atmosphere to change. Professional workers who are asked to advise on these matters need to explore previous relationships and new relationships with the spouse carefully before recommending living with the family rather than entering residential care. Above all, one must never 'take sides'. No coaxing to fulfil filial duty has much impact on this pattern. Parents very often feel closer to their children than the children do in return, and few parents and children confide in each other important decisions about key parts of their lives. It is best to direct efforts towards helping the elderly person accept the situation and develop alternative social supports.

(4) Problems created by the divorce of children. Divorce, formerly rare in the UK, is now so common that the divorce rate is the highest in Europe. It is often a major problem in the life of a parent and grandparent. In the first place, they often express the view that they have failed their children by not providing a satisfactory model of marriage as a basis for their children's marriage. Secondly, they find it difficult to adjust to the new lover or spouse while getting used to the break up of the old marriage, which is often sprung on them as a shock. Thirdly, and perhaps most difficult in may cases, is the removal of grandchildren, with whom a close love relationship has been built, as they move away with the divorced daughter-in-law or son-in-law.

(5) Hypochondriasis. Perhaps doctors find hypochondriasis difficult to tolerate. However, as age progresses, most individuals become more aware of their vulnerability and the need to take note of normal daily bodily functions, such as appetite, bowel function and sleep. This will include such common features as muscular pains and skin blemishes, so that it is not surprising that such concerns reach a peak in the elderly, for which they need reassurance. The experience of a stay in hospital is often disturbing, heightening the fear of dependence of others and the fear of death. These feelings are difficult to understand when you are under 40.

> A 77-year-old woman who lived alone and could not go out because of arthritis, was on our monthly visiting list. When calls were made, she was constantly abusive, refusing violently to be examined. She was clearly eating nothing but brown bread sandwiches and refused mobile meals and nursing care. An attempt was made to alter things by inviting the whole team to visit her, which made her furious and abusive to all. The only person she would tolerate was the young Home Help, who had two children. She spoke with bitter tears about the neglectful way her sons treated her and blamed their execrable wives for this.
>
> Eventually, the older son came to consult about his mother. It was pointed out that the mother felt bitterly that they had neglected her, and some cajoling took place to try to make him more aware of her need of the family. The reply was short and to the point, as he explained how, as children, he and his brother had been pushed outside the house for hours in all weathers when his mother had strange men in the house. They had nothing to repay her for.
>
> At this point, the Home Help left the service to spend more time with her two small sons. She was contacted and, because she was the only person who had made a relationship with the patient, agreed to continue to pay a daily visit, which she did until the patient had a stroke and died.

Anxiety in the elderly

The traditional view that old age is a time of peace and tranquility belongs to the age of the fairy story. The prevalence of anxiety is difficult to measure, but various studies produce figures of 15% in men and 30% in women, at ages between 65 and 80. There are three aspects, as at other ages: disturbance of mind, disturbance of body and disturbance of social behaviour. These vary from person to person, but there seems to be some consensus that the older person is more likely to complain of a disturbance of the body, rather than of the mind. There is a higher mortality rate, not explained by the presence of physical illness, in those with anxiety and depression compared with mentally well old people.

It is very important to distinguish those in whom anxiety has developed recently, from the life-long anxious person, who is more likely to have been sensitized to the danger of losing security as a result of an unpleasant childhood experience. The cause of recent anxiety may be social or biological, and can very often be remedied by the psychologically orientated physician.

Of the physical causes, the commonest causes of recent anxiety symptoms are cerebrovascular insufficiency and hyperthyroidism. Also, pulmonary embolism very often presents in the elderly as a sudden sense of apprehension, agitation and panic. It must be remembered that anxiety and depression, not only co-exist, but that depression may present as 'anxiety'.

It is always advisable to ask about self-administered drugs, including tea and coffee, because caffeinism may appear in an older person, not because of increased intake, but because tolerance to stimulants has decreased.

> A 79-year-old woman who had always been active, despite arthritic knees, began to lose weight and deteriorate generally. Full examination revealed no cause and she was admitted to hospital where extensive investigations failed to establish anything abnormal. A follow-up visit was arranged on discharge and half an hour was spent. This elicited that, in her parental home, there hung a list of couplets for every decade, of which she could remember none other than that for the 80-year-old woman, for apparently each sex was dealt with separately. It stated:
>
> 'Glued to her chair by weight of years
> She sits and waits till death appears.'
>
> This encapsulated memory, deeply impressed in childhood, had now been activated on reaching the age of 80. Discussion and demonstration of the gulf between the reality of that day and this enabled her to recover as mysteriously as she had become frail.

It has been suggested that there is a third reaction, other than fight or flight, in which the elderly 'freeze' and feelings are turned inwards for contemplation, reflection and acceptance.

Management of anxiety in the older person – Often isolated, the elderly are perhaps helped by talking and ventilating their feelings more than any other age group. Indeed, one can be less remote with older people, and unconditional positive regard for the patient and a correct understanding of the patient's situation open up the consultation. Techniques such as giving a full explanation of the medical condition, a specific organic diagnosis, providing treatment with the suggestion that he will improve within a certain time, is ineffective in the old. More is achieved by assuring the patient that he is indeed sick but that the physician will look after him. It is not wise to tell relatives that the patient's symptoms are psychologically based! And avoid responding to criticism of lack of interest by other doctors.

Drugs. In general, tranquillizers should be avoided, or used, if at all, for a limited period as one does with antibiotics. Diazepam is highly lipid soluble, and is distributed into lipid compartments more easily than in the young. Imipramine reduces anxiety extremely well, but, of course, tricyclics have cardiovascular and anticholinergic effects that limit their utility. I have often found 50 mg of Ascorbic acid given daily after psychotherapy a useful placebo.

Other methods. Old people may be helped by behaviour therapy, breathing exercises or group classes, and the well motivated can use the do-it-yourself tapes which can be purchased at many pharmacies.

DEPRESSION

The occurrence of mental depression increases with age particularly in postmenopausal women. Many aged persons regularly suffer from depression after exposure to stress. Those who have been in general practice, where most depressive illness is dealt with, will have noted that the onset of depression that is intractable to treatment and puzzling in origin often precedes malignant disease.

There is substantial evidence showing that depression is associated with an absolute or relative decrease in catecholamines, particularly in noradrenaline. At the same time, insufficiency of the central serotonergic processes may be one of the reasons for the high rate of anxiety and tension in depressed elderly people. Thus, both adrenergic and serotonergic functional depletion of the brain are important to the mechanism of depression.

Old patients rarely report depression for fear of advancing senility and mental illness, which may contribute to the low probability of recognition. But doctors also contribute by attitudes that suggest that old people are in an inevitable state of decline and that little can be done for them. Recognized early, depressive illness can be most successfully treated. It is important to distinguish clinical depression from the well-known features against the background which encourages old people to operate on the margins of society as second-rate citizens which may induce self reproach, and a sense of worthlessness.

There are those whose depressive episodes form a unipolar pattern, often associated with a positive family history. It is important to seek out, not only psychological reverses, but physical illnesses, such as pernicious anaemia etc., for it is to the general practitioner that the unique task of minimizing the impact of physical health on the prognosis of depression regularly falls. Impairment of physical health is the most important factor contributing to depression, and the most powerful predictor of outcome, particularly where there is pain, impaired mobility and restriction of the social role.

The tricyclic antidepressants, all of which come in 25 mg doses, are the mainstay of treatment. Amitryptilene, with a sedative effect, and imipramine for the lethargic have stood the test of time. Dothiepin and doxepin may be regarded as useful alternatives. They should not be changed until three weeks have passed (because the action is delayed) and should be continued for three to six months after recovery. The danger of cardiac arrhythmias is, in fact, low but should be borne in mind. Tetracyclic compounds have fewer side-effects, and are safe for those with cardiac damage. Their efficacy for depression, however, is no greater.

Psychological support is essential, either by the doctor or the community psychiatric nurse.

Referral is not often made, but those who should be referred are those who have made a suicidal attempt, or admit to planning to do so, and those with marked behavioural abnormality or psychopathology, with delusions or hallucinations, and those for whom home care seems inadequate. ECT is sometimes used for the very severe depressive with marked loss of function. The response of those with marked agitation is generally good.

INTELLECTUAL FAILURE

The majority of people undergo an inevitable decrement in certain mental faculties with age which arises from the interaction between intrinsic changes and the cumulative effect of injury and disease. Cognitive impairment is particularly evident where problems require rapid solution, due to delay within the central nervous system and sensorimotor slowing of the cerebral processes. Old people then find it more difficult to consider situations in new ways and settle into routines which encourage rigid mental states.

There is often impairment of memory, socially accepted in the forties to the extent that the forgetting of names is laughed about. However, the distinction between benign amnestic decay and early dementia is not clear.

Dementia does not conform to the norm for a disease process, being on a continuum between apparent normality and gross disturbance, depending on the stresses imposed and variation in the rate of its progression. The best way for the GP to regard these matters is to think of intellectual failure much in the same way that he considers cardiac failure. Dementia, like cardiac failure, is an end-point reached by many routes and results in disorganization of the personality. Whereas true dementia is irreversible (Alzheimer's disease), there are diseases, such as vitamin B_{12} deficiency, hypothyroidism, chronic subdural haematoma, normal pressure hydrocephalus, some endogenous psychoses, and space-occupying lesions, that can, in their earlier stages at least, be reversed.

Problems in the diagnosis of dementia

As in every other branch of medicine, there is no substitute for an adequate history and examination of the patient. The GP must be alert for the diagnosis of early cases, in order to plan ahead and to be able to instruct relatives. He will be confronted with the difficulty that subjects with a low score on memory and information tests nevertheless cope well with their environment and show little other intellectual deterioration. Many of these are subjects with low IQ and social class, and it is important to establish these facts early.

Language impairment

Language impairment is one of the central symptoms of dementia and the GP will be alert to poverty of expression, loss of ability to name objects and loss of fluency. This is so commonly accepted by relatives as a sign of old age that it is worth while employing tests of language function.

Mental testing

Whereas the young love to shine, old people fear to fail. Mental testing must, therefore, be introduced as part of the normal consultation. The Mental Status Quesionnaire has the virtue of being simple, yet with a high degree of discrimination. Its object is to test attention, memory, orientation and language. To use it, one does not have to be a clinical psychologist, and it can be carried out quite simply by relatively unskilled observers and it is acceptable to the patient. Remember that testing in the surgery may produce results very different from those obtained on the patient's home territory. The questions are:

- How old are you?
- What year were you born in?
- What is today's date?
- What month is it?
- What is the name of this place?
- What is the name of this town?
- Who is the Prime Minister?
- Who was the previous Prime Minister?

When the patient becomes aware of being tested, you may say: 'I am just wanting to see how good your memory is' and then, after discussing it, give a simple address, such as 57, St. James's Road, Wherever, stating that you will ask them later what it was. This provides a test of short-term memory.

There are many other tests of mental function. We have used the set tests successfully for years by simply asking people to name 10 objects, say colours, birds or towns. A man may like to be asked to name 10 football teams, and a woman 10 things that can be bought in the grocer's shop. If given four sets, then a score above 30 is acceptable, while those below 20 indicate probable dementia. It is interesting to note that, in each case, there will be hesitation, a stop, then one more object named before giving up, a finding which is quite consistent.

It is a good idea to carry out these tests before a member of the family, for the demonstration often produces the comment: 'Well, doctor, I never realized that he/she was quite so bad'. This assists in future planning.

Language function

Since vocabulary is often well retained despite a dementing process, it should be specially tested, both the ability to understand the spoken word and the ability to express language. Testing is done as follows:

(1) Simple commands (without gesture):
   i. Please sit down
   ii. Give me your coat
(2) Expressive aphasia:
   i. What is a refrigerator for?
   ii. What is a barometer for?
   iii. What is a thermometer for?
(3) Nominal aphasia:
   i. Ask the patient to name a wristwatch, strap and buckle, words which are in ascending order of unfamiliarity.
(4) Parietal lobe function (praxis and gnosia):
   i. Praxis: Touch your left ear with your right hand
   ii. Here are four matches. Please arrange them to make a square
   iii Gnosia: Name the coin in your hand (50p piece).

Finally, the ability to abstract may be done by asking the patient to say what well-known proverbs mean, bearing in mind the educational standard. There are degrees of complexity, of course, between 'look before you leap', 'a rolling stone gathers no moss' and even you, dear reader, may not find it easy to say what is meant by 'people who live in glass houses should not throw stones'!

Finally, always ensure that, if the results are poor, you are not dealing with a patient who is ill or tired. Investigations are then carried out, since 10–15% of patients have a cause that is treatable, and this will be important when the patient is referred.

Definition of dementia

Dementia remains a clinical description without any supposition about the underlying aetiology. Two main forms are described: senile dementia of the Alzheimer's type (SDAT) and multi-infarct dementia (MID). SDAT is perhaps more common in women and tends to be global eventually. Apraxia is an early sign, but memory loss precedes the other changes. Patients tend to be benign and bovine, often showing a shallow euphoria with some anxiety. However, few, if any, of the dementias are truly global, and most present with certain aspects of higher function more affected than others.

MID patients are more easily diagnosed, often being male with a history of recurrent strokes and the presence of unequivocal focal neurological signs. Difficulties arise when progressive intellectual failure is punctuated by one or more strokes of only mild severity. The deterioration is said to be stepwise, but is not always so. Unfortunately, some insight is often retained and emotional incontinence is a distressing feature of this illness. In the examination, particular attention is paid to the cardiovascular system, including chest X-ray and ECG. The treatment of those individuals with MID is along the same lines as that for completed stroke, with the aim of preventing recurrence, and control of hypertension, particularly systolic hypertension.

Management

Many patients are managed in the community. This involves an input of support for families and care for carers. Treatment of coexistent disease, e.g. infection or anaemia, is important. Aspirin and cerebral vasodilators may be used in MID. Cerebroactive substances are used empirically, for convincing evidence of reliable clinical improvement is lacking. Patients with this serious condition must be followed up regularly reassessed using the Clifton Assessment Procedure for the Elderly (CAPE) which provides scales for measuring the cognitive state and a behaviour rating. Measurement being fundamental to scientific enquiry the time has passed for intuitive diagnosis to suffice now there is daily contact with old people with mentally disabling disorders.

The future

The difficulty is that much has been written on advanced unequivocal cases. In practice, depressive symptoms often mask early dementia, or may confound it so that dementia is overdiagnosed. Mental tests can distinguish significantly between the normal and the demented, but early or borderline cases provide ambiguous results. Therefore, retesting is advocated but is time consuming. If it is delegated or referred to someone else, the clinical interview on which the diagnosis is based must first be standardized, ensuring that important symptoms are not forgotten by the interviewer and that his or her style does not colour the symptoms recorded. Some success has been reported showing that the Automated Geriatric Examination for Computer Assisted Taxonomy (AGECAT) compares favourably with the psychiatrist's diagnostic decision. It has no means as yet, however, of diagnosing most conditions needing exclusion, such as personality disorder and alcoholism. A short version, suitable for development in the community, of the Geriatric Mental State Examination (GMS) is being worked on.

There is, perhaps, an opportunity for prospective studies to begin in general practice with the cooperation of those working in departments of psychiatry.

At the moment, the problems inherent in these studies are extensive. The need for early diagnosis of senile dementia is clearly of great importance both to distinguish treatable from non-treatable causes so that treatment regimes may be implemented where appropriate, and to allow early implementation of promising treatments before gross behavioural changes have occurred. Dementia is, after all, the absolute indication for removing an old person from his home.

THE FEET

Probably no other part of the body reveals more clinical and social information in the elderly than the feet, where pulses, colour, temperature, trophic changes and oedema are all gathered conveniently into an accessible region. Circulatory impairment is associated with the formation of callosities, and other foot complaints with arthritis. Position sense, an absent flexor plantar response, and the ankle jerks, are all significant.

With age, the nails, for reasons unknown, become harder and thicker, and detritus is often found raising the great toe nail from its bed.

The loss of plantar fat pad, digital contractures, spur and hyperostotic formations, arthritic changes and functional adaptations are significant considerations in the development of hyperkeratotic lesions.

Modifications of shoes and footwear are important, and old people should be recommended the type of shoe which has a broad high toe box and wedge type of sole. Shoes should be chosen as late in the day as possible, as the feet swell gradually, and shoes purchased in the

> A 94-year-old lady was visited by the Health Visitor because she had been housebound for four years. It had been assumed that this was due to cardiac weakness, but inspection of the feet showed that there was considerable toe deformity, and walking was painful and unsteady. Surgical boots were ordered and the patient's name put down for a Rotary Club week at a new caravan near Selsey. The Rotarians considered her to be too old but eventually relented. During the week, the patient was taken to see a local market by car and asked if she could alight to look around. The volunteers were reluctant but allowed a short walk. This, in fact, took two hours, which exhausted them, but not the enthusiastic patient who lived on to be 100.

morning may pinch by late afternoon. The feet should be washed daily, and clean socks or stockings worn. Walking is the best exercise for the feet, and elderly females should be advised not to wear bedroom slippers throughout the day, but a court shoe with a low heel. Corns and calluses should be treated by a chiropodist, not cut at with a pocket knife or razor blade.

Further Reading

Murphy, E. (1986). (ed) *Affective Disorders in the Elderly*. (Edinburgh: Churchill Livingstone)

Brice Pitt. (ed) (1987). *Dementia*. (Edinburgh: Churchill Livingstone)

Wattis, J.P., Hindmarch, I. (eds.) (1988). *Psychological Assessment of the Elderly*. (Edinburgh: Churchill Livingstone)

Section 5
Society, Family and Community

AT RISK GROUPS

There are two basic ways of working in general practice. One is to study medical need in order to anticipate it and plan for it to be met; the other is to respond passively and defensively to symptom-orientated demand.

Studies have shown that only list size is strongly related to the components of work load, since a large list would be expected to contain larger amounts of need, with a higher level of demand for care, causing higher consultation rates and more contact time.

With regard to the elderly, a clear relationship exists between feeling overworked and the proportion of elderly patients for whom one is reponsible in a practice. The stress engendered by battling with problem solving in this group can generate defensive strategies, although different consulting patterns can result in different levels of unmet need. There can be no doubt that effectiveness and quality of care depend on factors other than the time and frequency of consultation. For instance, crowded waiting rooms, harrassed doctors, and 'busyness' may result in higher thresholds of entry to care, particularly for the elderly who are so often apologetic in their requests. On the other hand, the appreciation of potential and actual demand may produce modifications of work patterns that are within the control of a modern practice. For instance, in a very large authoritative study, general practitioners rated 62% of their time being occupied with trivial complaints. It is also clear that preventive programmes, encouraged by item of service fees for children and women of child-bearing age, are reflected in more doctor work for such groups, whereas loaded capitation fees have been seen as neither incentive nor adequate reward.

The elderly, as a group, have generally been regarded as unpopular for complex reasons. One major reason is that their complex medicosocial problems do not fit easily into the short consultation time that has become the norm in the NHS; another is because of a higher need for home visits at a time when these are falling generally. Above all, GPs become involved in crisis intervention in situations which it is often felt could have been avoided at the request of the distant relative paying an occasional visit at the week-end.

The planning of preventive care requires initial agreement and decision about method. This will include all members of the primary health care team, aided by volunteers, who can help with transport to surgery premises, and also, with some training, conduct interviews based on charts recording disability and health problems. The aim of such a scheme is simply to improve the quality of late life, rather than seek out occult threatening diseases which has been shown to be unproductive.

The team must decide on the age above which patients will be considered, and this will depend upon numbers. Perhaps the age 70 is ideal, but major problems usually develop in those over 75. The age/sex register is an essential tool. Patients may be selected if they have not been seen within a certain time. In the average practice, the number not seen during one year is about 18, and that not seen during the past six months is about 33 patients. We found that one quarter had not been seen because they were in excellent health and moving around independently, but, at the other extreme, we found isolation, depression, dementia, illiteracy and neglect.

In general, people are at risk when they live alone and are of advanced age. Then, there are those who have recently been discharged from hospital and those recently bereaved. Others are known with serious chronic illness and mental problems, especially those of a fluctuating course.

Caring for the elderly is placed in an entirely different perspective when all members of the primary care team cooperate in a programme to which all contribute. Patients can then be classified into three groups:

Group 1: Fully functional and independent,
Group 2: Function reduced by disability, requiring medication, special apparatus, and regular supervision for 'independence',
Group 3: Dependent patients, largely confined to the home.

The aim, which is very possible, is to move those from Group 2 into Group 1.

There are now many schemes described using postal questionnaires, visiting by a geriatric health visitor, street warden schemes, and other volunteers. Much of the methodology will depend upon whether the practice is inner city, urban/rural, suburban, compact or widely distributed. A movement which formerly involved only enthusiasts is now becoming common-sense good practice.

Living alone

This is not a simple issue. For instance, if living alone is regarded as a risk factor, the implication is that risks are removed when living with a family. However, living with others could produce delay in seeking help for a medical problem, whereas the cut-off point might be sooner when living alone.

Secondly, much depends on the personality of the individual. The GP will be in the advantageous position of knowing the patient's background. There are those, very often of schizoid temperament, who do not seek company and do not mix well. To them, the inner world of reality is infinitely preferable to the mess they see about them, and with which they find it difficult to compromise. Such people often live their lives in accordance with principles and a routine that gives them stability. On the other hand, there are those of a more cyclothymic temperament who are concerned with the feelings of others upon which they feed and depend. It is in this group that living alone gives rise to the dangers of isolation. The result here is that self neglect or self indulgence incur dangers; there is a feeling of loss and worthlessness which leads to depressive mood, the risk of alcoholism, or exploitation by others for the sake of company. When visiting such homes, one is often struck by the lack of discipline and untidiness, e.g. the 'depressed kitchen' with the draining board piled up with unwashed dishes.

There are cases where the health visitor can re-educate a patient in these circumstances. It is well known that widowed men return badly to the single status and respond well to a regular visit from a female member of the team who, while sympathetic, is firm in her expectations of what she will find on her next visit. Introductions to social groups and luncheon clubs are generally acceptable to this group, while other individuals respond well to the 'friendly visitor' who is, unfortunately for men who want to talk about football, usually female. Knowing about patients' interests will help, and I recall successfully introducing two ancient men who had fought in the first world war, which formed almost all their present conversation. A volunteer arranged to transport one to the other weekly, and eventually the local school referred pupils who were studying the 1914–1918 war to ask questions and take notes. Other arrangements may be successful in individual cases, for instance taking meals together. There are those who do not like luncheon clubs, but who remain interested in cooking and feel it is not worth cooking for one. It must be remembered that eating is still a social occasion for most people, despite the numbers one sees eating out of bags in the streets! New friendships can be made in this way, and table linen, long hidden away, is produced as part of the challenge of social intercourse, which raises standards and maintains social skills.

Then, there is the need, in some cases, to discuss residential care. The point here is that the decision must be made by the patient. The doctor may recommend it, and the social worker research the financial implications, what happens to furniture, and what type of accomodation will be most suitable. The fear in the minds of many old people is the 'unknown'. Therefore, no one should ever be removed to residential accommodation until they have seen it and approved of it. Nor should patients ever be sent into Part III or other accommodation on a social worker's report of inadequacy alone. A medical examination is essential.

Finally, it must be realized that one can still feel lonely in a group. I found this out in the same home which had 35 women residents and only three men. Of these three, one was very unhappy for no one understood that he was homosexual.

Retirement

Compulsory retirement at a given age is a modern phenomenon, for, 50 years ago, one half of the men over 65 were working. The age now chosen varies in different countries, but is becoming lower and is decided largely for administrative convenience rather than as a declaration of unfitness to continue in employment.

Retirement, therefore, has become one of the major psychosocial transitions in the lives of people, and is particularly stressful for males thought of as the 'head of the family' or the 'bread winner', especially in countries where the work ethic is strong. Thus, retirement is rated on the stress scale at 45%, not far below stresses such as bankruptcy, divorce and bereavement.

In women, adjustment is usually better because women undergo far more psychosocial transitions in life, whereas it seems that men simply gain their independence, and lose it. Thus women experience more stresses during puberty and courtship. When they marry, they usually change their name. It is they who bear the children, who menstruate and have a menopause. They face the empty nest situation more acutely, and then often re-enter employment, from which they then retire, and, finally, are far more likely to face bereavement and widowhood.

In recent years, the Pre-retirement Association has encouraged people to prepare for retirement, but this has largely appealed to middle class individuals to judge by the books on hobbies to be taken up, such as

> As medical officer to a local authority home, I paid a weekly visit to sort out any problems. I was asked, on one occasion, if I could help since a new patient was such a slow and untidy eater that a member of staff had to stay half and hour after all the other residents had gone to the common room. Examination showed that this patient had a Parkinsonian tremor and was overweight, with coarse features. TFTs confirmed myxoedema. Suitable treatment for both diseases solved the eating problem by 10 weeks, to the extent that the patient wanted to go home. It was a very sad moment when she had to be told that she no longer had a home to go to, as her family had sold it.

collecting china and making one's own sailing boat. General practitioners are often asked to lecture at these courses on health aspects, when they will stress diet, exercise, posture and human relationships.

Retirement is, therefore, a very individual matter and poor adaptation is common when not faced realistically. Industrial workers often feel 'put on the scrap heap', which induces depression and hours of boredom, sometimes embittered by waiting to see their mates emerge from the factory gates, but now as strangers. This encourages excessive smoking, increased alcohol consumption and gambling, shortening life expectancy. At the other end of the social scale, the man who has fulfilled important executive functions and has exalted status, is just as likely to languish in the void of retirement spent with a wife to whom he has become a stranger. For a man in the years following retirement, his status is largely maintained by the job he was doing.

The favoured life styles of retired people offer an understanding of male retirement:

(1) Continued interest and involvement in the work role as the main integrating factor in life.
(2) Increased engagement in family roles, spending more time with wife, grandchildren, and activities as a home-maker.
(3) Involvement in clubs, church, or civic/political activities. This type is seen where old people's clubs or campaigns are active in an area.

(4) The development of a former minor leisure activity or hobby into a major social role, such as gardening, collecting or travelling.
(5) A general reduction in the tempo of life, which continues much as before, with more time spent on non-work roles. This is perhaps the most common.
(6) Role-less activity, solitary passivity – watching TV, sitting by the window or in the park.

With improved health and financial status, retirement is gradually being viewed as a time of renewed opportunity. The transition time may span 5–10 years for some upper middle class professional people, and the general practitioner can provide much reassurance by offering a medical examination and counselling at this time. Even doctors have laboured under the false impression that the average survival time after the age of 65 was only two years compared with 12 years for those retiring at 60! The truth is that those retiring at 65 have an average life span thereafter of 14.1 years.

The age/sex register in my own practice contained the names of 16 men aged 64, two of whom had already retired on health grounds and two who intented working on after 65. A consultation proves useful in dispelling fantasies concerning retirement (one patient intending to spend every day fishing as he now did on Sundays).

Favourable features of the retired are:

(1) Happy marriage or its equivalent,
(2) Financial security,
(3) Community involvement with high status,

> I was visiting a 67-year-old man who had retired two years before as a bus driver. He had a younger wife, whose much younger sister had paid a visit and wanted to catch a bus home before dark. She asked her sister where the bus stop was, but, when she told her, the husband contradicted his wife and an argument broke out, during which the wife insisted she was right because she went shopping past the stop every day. At this, the husband rose to his full authority and declared: 'I ought to know: I used to do that route'. His humiliation became complete when he was told that the bus route had been altered six months previously.

(4) High educational standard,
(5) Previous good health based on good dietary habit,
(6) Absence of addiction to tobacco, alcohol, drugs or the sedentary life.

Preparation for retirement should commence at least five years before the event. Apart from matters of health, adaptation requires a very different life, usually involving assessment of house and neighbourhood. A large house can be costly to maintain and inconvenient in certain respects, e.g. electric points placed at ankle level, long staircases, many empty rooms, etc. A house is a machine for living in and heat insulation is an important point for older people. The role of the health worker is important in removing fantasies of retirement, and in helping to re-educate people in designing a second distinct life. Such fantasies are often based upon a happy holiday in the country or at a seaside resort. In some country towns, the suicide rate in the elderly is very high, and, in a famous seaside resort, problems may be caused when the husband dies within two years, and the wife cannot manage to climb up the hill from the shops near the sea front.

The problem faced by women retiring from work are not of the same order, for they assume domestic and social roles more easily and their status is based less on their former occupation.

Bereavement

Bereavement is the greatest crisis of late life, and it is then that it is most likely to be experienced. Despite its inevitability, few are prepared for it. If retirement is the crisis to be faced by men, widowhood is the lot of most women, who often begin rehearsing for it through spouse concern and speculation about the future in middle age.

The grief reaction, which is a subject in itself, is normally adjusted to in about twelve months and coincides roughly with the testamentary year for financial settlement. If patients have not passed through the usual process of numbness and disbelief, then anger and resentment, to depression and acceptance, the general practitioner may become involved with cases of depressive illness which are not easy to reverse. It is not unusual for males to have a resurgence of strong sexual feelings for which an understanding ear is all that is necessary.

However, in most cases, relationships have become habitual, based more upon a division of labour than upon emotional interchange. There

> An 81-year-old man was greatly upset by seeing his wife collapse and die from a stroke. He was supported through the grief reaction by the members of the team. Having been a professional soldier in earlier life, he showed remarkable capacity for self-care and discipline. It was debated whether he should be become a pensioner of Chelsea Hospital, but he decided against it. His house was poorly lit and cold in winter, and these deficiencies were rectified. He was much respected in the neighbourhood, repairing wireless sets and working in a large greenhouse, where he grew unusual flowers which he supplied to the ladies of the neighbourhood. He grew much of his own food in a small garden. He was prepared to endure loneliness, informing us that he had endured much worse when serving as a soldier far from home. When he was 90, his 56-year-old son's wife died from cerebral tumour, and the old man now had the job of comforting the son and preparing a meal when he returned from work. It was interesting to note how much the old man's functional capacity improved now he was needed to impart more than a father's comfort, but that of one who knew what the loss of a wife meant at first hand.

is no set pattern, but the loss of the physical and mental input of the dead partner into the domestic economy may easily lead to dependency on, and sometimes exploitation by, unscrupulous relatives. It is perhaps wise, therefore, for older people to learn how to do the household finances, to shop and to cook, in preparation for the time of widowhood.

The best support can be given by a general practitioner who has understood the life of the family prior to the death of the spouse. It is not always good for 'Mum' to be taken away by the children until she has adapted to some extent. The continuing running of the home is a priority, and sensitivity to the old person's wishes, which are not always verbally expressed, is needed.

The bereaved must be helped towards autonomy and independence. The worst thing that can happen is a takeover. An occupational therapist may well be asked to assess performance of the activities of daily living, and a social worker may well advise on financial and legal aspects. The general practitioner who offers a physical examination at this time is acting most appropriately, since old people often doubt their capacity to carry on alone. Modifications to the home may be suggested at this stage, and should be speedily provided where dependency is threatened.

CULTURAL ASPECTS

Attention is increasingly paid to cultural factors in what is now a multiracial society. This works both ways. The public school demeanour of the British GP can produce lack of understanding when dealing with Asian patients, and doctors with strong retention of Asian culture may have difficulty in comprehending matters that go without saying among the native British. For instance, looking someone straight in the eye is regarded in traditional British culture as a sign of honesty and trustworthiness, and not to do so is thought 'shifty'. On the Indian subcontinent, however, one is taught that the reverse applies, for respect and politeness require the gaze to be averted. Major aspects, such as circumcision rites and the practice of purdah by Muslim women in the presence of men, are generally recognized, but the time is approaching when larger numbers of older people will swell the ageing population from immigrant groups.

This is a very large subject, but only one or two main points will be considered.

In Asian communities, the elderly are important members of extended families, respected, wanted and loved. They play a large, and sometimes dominant, part as culture protectors, nurses and child minders. It is not uncommon for the whole family to bring a sick relative or child to the consultation and for the grandmother to act as spokesperson. The elderly expect to be employed until they die, a feature of the agricultural and naturalistic societies of origin. There is a strong leaning to self medication and the avoidance of certain meats. Thus, an elderly patient of Asian origin may complain of feeling very weak, having eaten karela, an Indian vegetable which lowers blood sugar and can produce prolonged hypoglycaemia in conjunction with chlorpropamide.

Religious convictions run deep and should be respected. Elderly Muslims may travel back to Mecca, and Indians return to India to renew their faith, encountering health hazards, such as bovine tuberculosis, malaria, amoebic dysentery, or poisoning by holy foods which have not been refrigerated during return. Care must be taken in discussing matters upon which strong views are held by ethnic Asians, such as euthanasia, for, where British patients may be impressed and even guided by rational morality, strict religious observance governs the Asian mind.

Patience must be shown with elderly relatives who come as visitors. Western ways of life often cause culture shock, the most extreme example of which is perhaps the cultural taboo on parts of the body such as the anus, genitalia and feet. Rectal examination must, therefore, be preceded by sometimes lengthy counselling. This also includes medication given by the anal and vaginal routes, including, of course, enemata. The left hand is used for cleaning such parts, and therefore, a nurse may be required for fitting ring pessaries and changing them. There is considerable value in the practice having a female partner where Asian patients are concerned, and, in matters of difficulty, much help can be obtained by local community leaders, local priests and voluntary organizations. It is a very good idea to have the practice policy written in various languages for patients with a rudimentary knowledge of English.

The Caribbean elderly are fewer in number at present, but it is worth noting that negro women are less likely to suffer from osteoporosis. Arcus senilis is, however, seen frequently in negroes in their middle forties. Hypertension is more common in negroes, but it is not established whether this is a racial characteristic or due to the increased stress of adaptation to a harder life in Britain.

Finally, it must not be overlooked that there are strong codes concerning the dying, so that a non-Muslim should only touch the body of a deceased Muslim with gloves, in order not to defile it before the priest has visited.

There are also considerable regional variations of culture in the British Isles, with which a doctor should establish an early knowledge when seeking a practice outside the area of his own upbringing. These are now more concerned with speech and idiom than with custom, but it is not long since that women in South Wales mining areas did not attend the funeral of their husbands for economic reasons clearly understood there. Neither can a Hindu woman attend the funeral of her husband, but must wait with her in-laws and family whose duty it is to look after her.

INSTITUTIONALIZATION

Increasingly, GPs are looking after elderly people in residential, nursing and rest homes for the elderly. When the possibility of removal from home to an institution arises, the decision-making process is one of the most delicate situations in which the GP is involved. In many cases, admission to hospital, in emergency or because of irreversible mental failure, causes no problems. It is when a combination of medicosocial factors, such as frailty, poverty and unsuitable housing, occur, often stressed by family or neighbours, that decisions have to be made.

Older people and their families suffer intensely when removal from home becomes necessary. The old person experiences anxiety, fear and a sense of rejection and abandonment, while family members have painful emotions of guilt, conflict, sadness and shame. Well-meaning anxious families may deny the patient the opportunity to participate in this decision to the fullest extent possible. At the least, the patient should be fully informed about the options being considered and carefully prepared for any change contemplated.

What is particularly trying for old chronically ill patients is the likelihood of being transferred several times from the community to an institution, or from one institution to another. The harmful effects can, to some extent, be mitigated by correct referral in the first instance after a full examination and assessment. Perhaps the most awkward mistake is referring a confused patient to a psychiatrist when the patient has in fact a pneumonic infection without fever. Most patients, however, will be fully aware of what is happening and should be given the opportunity to manipulate their institutional environment. All too often, they are run along boarding school lines, in situations where periodic in-service training and support is not provided for the staff. GPs can often make recommendations in these circumstances. A sense of hopelessness if often felt when patients fear that eventual discharge is unlikely. Arrangements can often be made for such individuals to be looked after at week-ends and for other short periods by the family.

Most doctors will have observed with revulsion homes where, through congregated living, institution-orientated activities, removal of personal property, involuntary incarceration under constant observation, and no promise of release, patients undergo rapid deterioration, sitting around the walls staring into space, as if waiting for transport to eternity. GPs who visit such institutions will note the withdrawn patient, sitting in a flexed posture, apparently unaware of her surroundings, but surprisingly obedient to command. This is rarely the fault of the staff, who are kept busy with dressing, feeding, cleaning etc.

It must be remembered also that 'institutionalization; can occur to varying extents in old people living in their own homes, and in families when they perform scheduled activities under constant observation, within a kind of standardized sanction system where no decision making is required.

It is a general feeling that voluntary organizations succeed better than public authorities in providing atmosphere and opportunities for individuality and personality to flourish. They are likely to have less rigidity and conformity to externally imposed rules and thus, a better chance to adapt to the needs of the people within them. If there is some truth to such generalizations, there are examples of good, bad and indifferent homes in each type of establishment. Voluntary organizations may be more selective in allocating places, and private homes need to satisfy commercial as well as welfare interests, while local authorities must meet the whole range of needs presented to them, which are not otherwise met.

A new generation of elderly people is now coming to need residential accommodation with expectations based on previous experience of higher living standards, better education, and less acquiescence in what others order for them. There will be expectations of single rooms, private washing and toilet facilities, personal furniture and opportunity for continuing social interests.

While there is a natural desire not to segregate people, there may be a limit to the tolerance which can reasonably be expected of those old people whose mental state and behaviour is extremely distressing to others with whom they share a home. This is no easy matter to resolve, for old people should not be shunted from home to home as they get older, change and deteriorate. Planned policies may well be over-ridden by the increasing pressure upon homes to relieve urgent problems elsewhere. Shortage of places creates pressures which reduce the standard of care and remove from old people and their families the freedom of choice. Moving into residential accommodation must not mean moving out of the life once known.

HOUSING

For most old people, the home is a love object and a time capsule, enshrining its saga of the relatives who have lived there, a symbol of family unity and tradition. Many old people in a practice have lived for more than thirty years, and some for more than sixty, in the same house. Very often, the house has become entirely unsuitable for the present incumbent; having once housed a family, it is now too large for safety and comfort, with many empty rooms and neglected fabric.

Very often the neighbourhood has changed and the concentration of elderly people reduced. Much depends on the physical environment and the borders of the cognitive neighbourhood, defined very often by street slopes, heavy vehicular traffic, convenience shopping, and the demarcation of racial characteristics and socio-economic status.

While one cannot change a neighbourhood, modifications of the home must be considered. The idea is often advanced that old people are happiest when left in their own homes, and that to move them is a recipe for disaster. This may have been true before there were the attractive alternatives of specially-built homes with their obvious convenience. To a new generation of old people more used to social mobility, moving is often a great success. Although the matter is usually referred to a social worker to work out details, it is the GP who estimates, in the first place, whether the home may be converted, for example by bringing the bed downstairs or constructing a toilet nearby for those finding it difficult to reach the upper floor. This enables the upper floor to be let, thereby increasing income and providing some supervision and a sense of security. Sometimes a person's entire capital is locked up in their property, so that their income remains insufficient for heating and feeding. Modifications that might be needed concern:

1. Heating: safety of appliances, e.g. heat guards, flues, electrical installations, switches, wires. The need for extra heating to achieve the minimum safe temperature of 18.3°C.

2. Economy: reduction of heat loss, insulation.

3. Lighting
   (a) Illumination where it is most needed, e.g. staircases, over sinks, in cellars and porches, and outside where there are steps and garbage disposal areas.

(b) Installation: Old premises may need rewiring or there may be a fire hazard. Where plugs are inserted and removed frequently, it is helpful to position them at waist height.

4. Ventilation: This is often poor when old people take up their quarters in a small room in which doors and windows are barricaded against heat loss. Carbon dioxide levels increase, producing drowsiness. The old-fashioned fire place, still often used, assisted ventilation by drawing air in to the room, but a gas or solid-fuel appliance needs an outlet to prevent carbon monoxide levels building up.

5. Fire hazards: Old people become less aware of their surroundings through impaired vision and reduced sense of smell. They need to be reminded of fire hazards and to take precautions.
   (a) To use a lighter rather than matches,
   (b) To avoid smoking in bed, or in armchairs if likely to fall asleep,
   (c) To install a fire extinguisher and to inform neighbours where it is,
   (d) Not to store inflammables, such as turpentine, indoors,
   (e) To buy flame-resistant night clothes and chair covers,
   (f) Never to carry heaters from room to room, to install them against the wall away from cross draughts, to have heaters serviced regularly, and to be careful when filling them.

6. The bedroom: The position of this room is all important. A trial period of sleeping downstairs will often persuade reluctant old people of the benefits when there is heart disease for which stair climbing is an aggravating factor. The height of the bed needs to be considered, for old people find it easier to get in and out of a high bed rather than a low one. A mattress that is too soft makes these manoeuvres difficult. An electric overblanket, provided it is absolutely safe, is an important means of maintaining even body warmth.

7. The bathroom: The dangers to guard against are falling, slipping, scalding and electrocution.
   (a) Have a handrail placed vertically beside the bath.
   (b) Most modern baths have non-slip surfaces. If not, a special mat may be purchased from hardware stores that is held down by suction pads.
   (c) A bath seat is important for those with frail or arthritic limbs who cannot sit right in or get out of the bath by kneeling.

(d) The temperature of the bath water should always be tested before entering.
(e) The presence of an electric heater is to be discouraged.

8. The toilet: Important points to consider have already been dealt with in the section on Incontinence (q.v.).

REFERENCES

How, NM. (1973). A team caring for the elderly at home. *J R Coll Gen Practit*, **23**, 627-636

Qureshi, B. (1986). Management of ethnic Asian patients in general practice. In Pereira Gray, DJ. (ed.) *The Medical Annual*

Section 6
Uses of . . .

USES OF DRUGS

The elderly patient is perhaps better able to benefit from wise drug therapy than any other age group because old age is the time when deficiencies occur, so that most satisfying responses are seen when replacement therapy is used, as in pernicious anaemia, thyroid deficiency, senile vaginitis, Parkinson's disease and hypokalaemia. No less impressive is the action of tricyclic drugs in depressive illness and the use of corticosteroids in the control of giant cell arteritis.

On the other hand, drugs have a limited role in the treatment of many elderly people who are better served by attention to their social environment and physical therapies. Unfortunately, for too many, the administration of drugs has become synonymous with treatment. In old age, where so many deviations from health can be identified and, as it were, 'treated', there is a real threat of iatrogenic harm. 87% of patients over 75 take regular medication, and 1 in 4 take regimes of three or four drugs. Doctors are doubtful about compliance and it is remarkable that drugs are still given to patients who can neither read nor understand the instructions, and who are undergoing self medication with indigestion and cough medicines, laxatives, etc. Unless one is in general practice, it is impossible to know how difficult it is to move in the direction of precision and control. The pharmacology of geriatrics has lagged behind many other aspects of that discipline, with the result that pharmacotherapy remains an art, based more on intuition and personal experience than upon scientifically substantiated facts.

Factors affecting drug action in the elderly

The picture of the vulnerable individual is one with multiple pathologies, a small lean body mass, impairment of mental function, some degree of liver or kidney damage, and a possible previous adverse reaction to a drug.

With advancing age, there is some impairment of active and passive absorption due to changes in the intestinal mucosa, alteration in blood flow, and rising pH of gastric contents. Other factors include alteration in gastric emptying, with decreased intestinal motility and fewer cells available for absorption.

The finding of higher plasma levels, on the other hand, is due to other altered processes, such as reduced rate of elimination or distribution of a drug. After all, older people are, on average, smaller, and total body water and lean body mass are reduced, while decreasing cardiac output results in a smaller proportion of the blood flow entering the liver and kidneys. Protein binding is altered due to a lowered plasma albumin level, which affects such drugs as carbenoxalone and phenytoin. The increase in percentage of body fat, especially marked in women, means that highly lipid-soluble compounds can become increasingly localized in body fats, so that there is increased duration of action or reduced concentration in the blood. The duration of action of highly lipid-soluble drugs is determined by their metabolism to an inactive form for excretion by the kidneys. Thus, the plasma half-life of paracetamol is prolonged in the elderly, especially in those who are slow metabolizers. Higher nitrazepam levels persist in slow acetylators. This difficult area for clarification has to be considered against environmental factors, such as smoking, alcohol intake, and the effects of other drugs given concurrently. We must also remember that there are changes in the sensitivity of receptor sites.

Most ageing organs have reduced ability to respond to stress and there is less flexibility to changes induced by drugs. Thus, drugs acting on the myocardium may bring about a lower response because of the increased percentage of fibrous tissue found in cardiac muscle. Digoxin, for instance, and the aminoglycoside antibiotics are excreted by glomerular filtration at a rate that correlates with it. Penicillin, on the other hand, is secreted by the renal tubule. High drug levels can then occur as a result of impaired renal functions. Nor must it be forgotten that the accessory excretory function of the skin is almost negligible in most old patients who are particularly liable to further impairment from other factors, such as dehydration, congestive cardiac failure, hypotension, urinary retention, and parenteral damage from diabetic nephropathy.

Helpful guidelines in prescribing

First of all, is drug therapy required at all? Many regimes can be pruned and drugs avoided by discussing altered life styles and by allaying anxieties. The GP will then find himself using only those drugs which are really needed and of which he fully understands the action.

When considered necessary, drugs should be prescribed in minimal numbers, beginning with the lowest possible dosage, so reducing the chance of incompatibilities and making it easier to track down the agent responsible for any side effects that may occur. Above all, if we use a limited number of drugs, it becomes easier to be sure how a drug is metabolized and excreted, and this may prevent accumulation which, with hypotensive agents, for instance, leads to the danger of falling.

Many group practices now limit their prescribing to an agreed list of drugs.

Treatments should be reviewed frequently to prevent drugs on repeat lists being continued longer than is necessary.

The aim should always be one of short term therapy and drugs should be used like antibiotics – carefully selected and prescribed with a definite course in mind.

Once daily dosage aids compliance, though combinations should be avoided except to facilitate the lowest possible dosage.

Identify those who will need help with compliance.

Whenever new symptoms are advanced, therapy should be reviewed, and direct enquiry made about self-medication. This includes, not only those drugs which may be purchased over the pharmacy counter, but also drugs supplied from other patient's stores!

Practical suggestions

(1) Containers. This aspect is of special importance in dispensing practices, but is not confined to them. Medicine bottles should be large enough to be easily handled, and the neck wide enough to allow easy flow of the contents. The top must be capable of being removed with ease, which means that childproof lids, which present difficulty to many frail hands, should be issued only to old people living with children. Bubble packs are also not easy for patients with reduced manual dexterity.

(2) Clarity. Compliance is not simply obtained by obedience to a command! There must be a clear exposition by the prescriber and a clear understanding and agreement by the patient. Vague instructions like 'to be taken as directed' went out with plus fours and musical evenings.

(3) Coping with tablets. Some cannot manage large tablets, while others cannot manage small ones. Oval tablets are more easy to take than round ones, and tablets are less likely to stick on the way down than capsules. Transit is aided by swallowing in the upright position with a drink of at least 100 ml water.

(4) Combination products. These may aid compliance and should be used when a single drug is inadequate. Careful monitoring of say potassium levels when prescribing thiazides with potassium sparing agents is still required, and these principles take priority over cost benefit considerations.
(5) Culprits, or drugs commonly producing unwanted effects in the elderly. Confusiogenic drugs are, of course, centrally acting and include hypnotics, tranquillizers and antidepressants, but also anticholinergics and anti-Parkinsonian drugs, such as levodopa and bromocriptine. We may add to this list anticonvulsants, and the hypoglycaemic effect of drugs used in Type II diabetes. Others to consider are digitalis glycosides and corticosteroids. NSAI drugs and cimetidine. Some of these drugs will be responsible for postural hypotension, but the chief culprits are all the antihypertensives. They must be considered in cases of falls, and also carbamazepine, phenytoin and glyceryl trinitrate. It is well known that antipsychotic drugs may produce parkinsonism, yet it is still found that prochlorperazine has been prescribed for 'giddiness' when a moment's reflection would make it clear that an antipsychotic drug can do no good and may do harm. We are left with a long list of drugs, led by codeine, which may produce constipation. Nor must we overlook the diuretics which may cause constipation and dehydration, but can produce urinary incontinence and, occasionally, have goutogenic and diabetogenic effects.

Finally, the harmful effects of the drug Opren were first noted among elderly patients but the warnings were not heeded at first. This will remind those of us who prescribe for old patients that they are more sensitive indicators of adverse effects.

USE OF THE TEAM

The team as a whole

Whether formulated or not, each practice has policies. Modern practice is generally orientated heavily toward health promotion and prevention of illness. The team approach arose out of the wide scope and interdisciplinary cooperation required by geriatric medicine, and, increasingly, the care of the elderly in general practice is taking its place alongside paediatrics, family planning, hypertension screening and other activities.

Attachment schemes mean that the integrity of a team is difficult to maintain over a course of several years, due to changes. In some instances, interference in its action from senior officers of paramedical disciplines outside the practice undermine activities. Health visitors are, at present, encouraged to include the elderly in their surveillance, alongside mothers and babies.

While multidisciplinary care is widely admired as a means of delivery of care, hardly any studies of evaluation have taken place. The composition of the practice population will be a determining factor of the way the team is composed and the way it operates.

Team function

This can be stated as follows:

(1) To cover all patients at risk by selection from an age/sex register.
(2) To survey at-risk groups continuously.
(3) To step in at the right time (crisis prevention and intervention).
(4) To promote health by education and screening.
(5) To reduce pressures of illness and environmental stress.

The formulation of objectives

Unless the team sets itself objectives it cannot assess its results or monitor its performance.

A model

The use of the team by Dr Normal How was an excellent model. Old patients' records were kept in an open file in four sections, one each for the doctor, nurse, health visitor and social worker. Each of these team members visited the patients in their section once in eight weeks, which meant that the patient received a fortnightly visit from team members in succession. This was a routine with inbuilt flexibility, since if, for instance, the social worker thought that the patient's health had deteriorated, she would place the card in the doctor's section of the file, perhaps marked 'urgent'. The health visitor, on the other hand, might consider the patient needed more advice on heating allowance, and would break the succession by putting the card back in the social worker's section, and so on. In this way, the team maintained its pulse on the elderly section of the practice efficiently, and notes were shared.

USE OF THE HOSPITAL

The essence of the practice of geriatric medicine in hospital consists of the basic ingredients of acute medicine, rehabilitation and long-term care, together with the day hospital and community involvement. The ways these elements are compounded vary widely according to the history of the department and the philosophy of the consultants. Some have all their beds on one site and serve a dense population in a small area, but others may have beds in several hospitals spread over rural areas of considerable area. Some have inherited a tradition of receiving most patients from other clinicians, whereas others have established their own direct admissions, and have developed where there has been a shortage of general medical or psychiatric facilities. Some have acute, rehabilitation and long-term patients in each ward, but, in most hospitals, these are separate functions. In country districts, small community hospitals exist where GPs can admit elderly patients, with consultant availability. This is an excellent system.

The aim is to return as many patients as possible to the community. Standards of care are usually measured by the length of bed occupancy, but this depends on assessing the resources available, such as the provision of domestic help, the provision of meals, and the continuing provision of medical and nursing care. Some of these functions are efficiently transferred, but others fail because of lack of input resources. Other standards are equally, or more, important, such as the recreation unit activities, which may include classical music, a debating society, cookery, handicrafts and beauty groups which exist in some hospitals, while, in others, all long-stay patients sit in geriatric chairs in their night clothes.

How far is the hospital a community resource?

With 94% of people over the age of 65 living outside institutions (Britain has the highest rate of any country in this respect), much medical and social care inevitably falls upon those providing primary care. Difficulties occur in two areas:

(1) Crisis intervention. There is an ever-present need for back-up beds to be held in readiness for emergency admission. At times when this resource is most likely to be needed, it is usually lacking because of increased pressure on bed capacity.
(2) High-dependency care. The more efficient the primary care team becomes in maintaining people in the community, the greater the

number of highly dependent patients that are generated, so that an uneasy balance exists between the input of medical and nursing resources and the containment of the problems.

When and what to refer

Emergencies are sent to the appropriate special department, e.g. acute abdomen to general surgery, and acute glaucoma to ophthalmology.

The GP, however able, gets stuck at times. The patient lives alone and has mobility problems within the home. The GP has found a number of conditions, but is unable to explain the falling haemoglobin level. Here, a 24-hour admission is an efficient way of helping the patient and the GP.

The domiciliary consultation enables the consultant and GP to meet at the home. He is unlikely to suggest the 'correct' diagnosis, but it is important that he should assess the home to which the patient will return, if admitted. Some geriatricians bring their team, nurse, sister, occupational therapist, physiotherapist and social worker, with them, on occasions.

Referral to outpatients is more common, and is the gateway also to the day hospital.

What to say

Good communications are very important, and are aided when the consultant knows the practice and the practitioner understands the facilities and the problems faced by hospital colleagues.

The referral letter should state clearly why the referral is being made, and what the practitioner expects from the consultation. Most important, the patient's background should be stated, and such information as previous occupation, previous medical history, marital status and next of kin, should be stated. Relevant investigations should be detailed, and something may be added about the patient's interests and motivation. Sometimes a telephone call will save time and enable the features of an individual to be conveyed in a few minutes.

Investigations

It is perhaps in the elderly that the fullest use of investigation can be made. But this is only possible when there is a collection service from the practice centre to the laboratory. Otherwise, it is best to arrange for the patient to go to, or to be referred to, the outpatients department.

The use of radiology is also important, not only in fractures, but in estimating cardiothoracic ratio for heart enlargement, distinguishing between forms of arthritis, and Looser's zones in the chest, osteoporosis in the spine, and examining for the presence of bony secondaries.

The day hospital

This is not to be confused with day centres. The day hospital is the logical evolution of the geriatric hospital providing a bridge with the community it serves. Patients should be referred only when there are good opportunities for rehabilitation. The GP should visit the local day hospital in order to know what it offers. It is of interest and also educational to watch ADL assessments, instruction in the use of aids, and to see several occupational therapists at work. Of particular interest is seeing patients, for whom life had been a matter of grim endurance, now cheerfully chatting over a meal in bright surroundings. Fear of hospital, which is common in the elderly, is often removed by such experiece. The difficulty is, of course, the question of turnover, which limits the introduction of new cases.

A final point is to stress the importance of visiting the discharged patient early, for readaptation is often difficult.

USES OF PRACTICE CLINICS

The most valuable use of team resources can be made by using practice premises for special clinics.

Assessment clinics

These are sometimes run by health visitors. Patients are weighed and measured, and have their urine tested and blood pressure taken. Problems with vision and hearing are considered, and, in some instances, mental testing is carried out. Using a questionnaire, a small proportion of patients are referred to the GP, or followed up by other team members. Very often, the GP sets aside a special session and is present, carrying out medical examination.

Clinics for special groups

Some centres covering more than 20,000 patients find it useful to have a Stroke Club. This, in fact, may grow to include other forms of handicap. Patients and their principal helpers are invited. Talks can be given by each member of the team, describing the role of each. At the end, question-and-answer session over a cup of tea reveals many misunderstandings and rectifies omissions. Above all, it reveals the importance of caring for the carer, for many of whom it may be their only outing, and who feel generally isolated to the extent that they have emotional problems themselves. Transport can often be arranged by the Lions or Rotary Club.

Many other groups can be arranged – for instance, a session for grandmothers who feel useless because the health visitor has become the recognized authority figure in the upbringing of young children.

I found, in my practice, that there were many children who had no grandmother, who is a very important figure, while there were some spinsters, who had not married because of past misfortune, but loved children. With the help of other team members, introductions were made, to enable grandmothers to be 'adopted' with mutual benefits.

The use of surveillance

Whatever one's view of formal screening programmes, there can be little doubt of the importance of surveillance of the elderly. Patients are reassured by it: crisis intervention is often prevented. In most practices, 98% of the community nurse's visiting list consists of patients over the age of 70, so that a daily meeting is, for most practices, the main method of surveillance. Other cases come to light from members of the 'extended' team, for instance when a minister of religion reports illness in one of his parishioners, or the milkman expresses concern about a client becoming frail or failing to collect her milk. Some practices send postcard questionnaires to patients on their birthday, and respond to answers indicating decline.

There are two areas where surveillance is important for the GP. Firstly, he can train himself to do a quick screen on every old patient who enters his consulting room. This would involve observing the gait, the dress, facial expression, the manner of sitting down, the corners of the mouth, and the manner and matter of speech, from each of which much can be derived. Secondly, a regular review of the repeat prescription list is necessary every three months, or at least a review of the individual, who could be handed a questionnaire concerning the effects of drugs and the way they are managed.

USE OF DAY CENTRES, COMMUNITY CLINICS

There is, in Britain, a clear distinction between part of the hospital service, the geriatric day hospital, and the provision, by the local authority social services department, of social day centres, staffed by social care givers and volunteers. There is some overlap in some areas where there is joint funding, and where medical and other assessments are performed by professionals at day centres. Some day centres are focussed on church premises which may make non-church attenders feel excluded. There seems to be a sharp division between those who are clubbable and those who are not. The small grey area in between may relieve isolation and monotony for a few. Depending on local organizers, a variety of activities are undertaken, including old time dancing, exercise sessions, playing games, and going on coach outings. Perhaps recruitment is particularly useful to an elderly person who moves into the area without knowing anyone. GPs may be asked to give talks on health, and be embarrassed to find that just after he has finished unsuitable buns, heavily buttered, and cakes are brought in and despatched with voracity by an audience that is noticeably overweight!

Community clinics are sometimes set up in a district by health visitors to promote health education among older people. These are usually very well organized, with posters and literature prominently displayed. Occasionally, a local GP with a special interest will attend, but difficulty may arise when asked to see other doctors' patients. They are not always popular when cases have to be referred to practitioners of the type who would rather 'let sleeping dogs lie'. It would be more efficient if health visitors were given the opportunity to conduct these services from general practices.

USE OF VOLUNTEERS

Medical care is a small part of the total care of the elderly, which involves an extensive and varied social dimension. Social workers are concerned with factors which might include: accommodation, financial problems, the physical and/or mental condition of the client, problems experienced by the client's family, isolation, adequacy of support from relatives and/or existing services, the notion of 'risk', precipitating events, and pressures exerted by other services. In many areas, there is a lack of service availability and delivery, and many practices do not have social work attachment. However, pathways through services are determined, not only be availability, but by alternatives. Furthermore, studies of the general practitioner referral process show that doctors vary greatly in referral practices.

Linkage with volunteer groups seem to be an important development for practice centres. We found that 200 voluntary workers, attached to a local church, ran a 'pop-in' club which relieved loneliness and alerted organizers to cases of special need. They were invited to work in the Health Centre two mornings a week. Among their activities are: providing transport, a street warden scheme, provision of information, leaflets, etc., replacement of hearing aid batteries, friendly visiting, 'granny sitting', etc. and a variety of needs, such as the old lady who had removed her curtains and washed them, but was afraid she might fall in the more difficult job of replacing them. She contacted the centre and a volunteer went back to the house with her. Other elderly people have received help with garden work from youthful volunteers.

It is important to realize that a kind heart and willingness are not enough, and education classes and a booklet on common problems help to raise the standard. Thus, street wardens are able to recognize home hazards and to take steps to prevent hypothermia in winter for those at risk in the street. Use of emergency call devices is also proposed: the Weyrock system (now out of date in our area) illuminates a 'HELP' sign in the window, and the police ensure that a Panda car patrols a number of streets with wardens once every night.

Some important research projects in general practice would not have been possible without the recruitment of volunteers to help with distribution of questionnaires and clerical work.

Finally, we should constantly remind ourselves that the Home Help Service and the Mobile Meals Service began as ideas in the minds of female voluntary workers.

Section 7
The Whole Person

THE WHOLE PERSON

The concept of whole person care is important at every age. It is particularly so in older people living in times very different from those of their formative years, and perhaps experiencing disintegration of the personality.

To address them, therefore, as 'Gran' or 'old fellow' will reinforce the lost sense of personal identity and convey them to a featureless limbo, rather then keep them as a member of the most varied of all age groups.

Perhaps those caring for the elderly should be among the best educated members of their profession, able to communicate beyond clinical situations about the novels of Wells, Kipling, Gissing and Conrad, or the politics of Asquith, Bonar Law and Lloyd George?

How did early training, with an easier acquaintance with death but a taboo on sex, influence their development?

What sort of family nurtured them? It would almost certainly be larger than families are today, and perhaps only present in photographs.

How do they feel in a world where most things are openly practised but were against the public morality of their early years?

How have they adjusted – by acceptance, anger, criticism or apathy?

What have been their previous occupations? How has this influenced their health? Having, perhaps, struggled hard with little to show, how do they feel about the affluence enjoyed by many young people today?

Where have they lived; at home or abroad? How long have they lived in the practice area? Have you visited the home, for, unless you have, how can you call yourself a 'family' doctor? Or are you just a technocrat?

What illnesses have they had in the past, and how have they coped? These questions are worth asking the young doctor who may think all old ladies are 'look-alikes', with glasses, short stature and white curly hair.

WHAT ARE THE AIMS OF CARE OF THE ELDERLY?

The elderly have no different needs from any other age group: good health, happiness, nourishing food, warmth, suitable housing, self-respect, the affection of others, and the occasional luxury.

Behind the well-known epigram giving the aim of geriatric medicine: 'give life to the years, not years to the life' is the serious implication that it is not humane to create forms of medicated survival. Many instances will be met in which clinical wisdom is placed above clinical knowledge. The team is responsible for:

1. Preventive measures;
2. Checks on development;
3. Appropriate management of common disorders;
4. Full assessment; physical, social and psychological;
5. Planning care in accordance with prognosis and diagnosis;
6. Recognizing the importance of the crises of late life, and preparing for retirement, bereavement and the patient's own death;
7. Taking steps to prevent crisis intervention, but ready to step in when needed?
8. Teaching, communicating and training the elderly in self care and independence; and
9. Making use of every service, statutory and voluntary, with the aim of slowing biological ageing, and hence concomitantly the various diseases of ageing.

WHO IS INVOLVED?

Levels of care

(1) Self care. This can often be taken for granted in the elderly, but may be pushed too far with resultant neglect. Time is well spent teaching old people the role of each team member and how to deal with common problems, such as insomnia, the desire for self medication, etc.

(2) Primary professional care is the care that provides first contact and, often, long-term continuing care. These include:
   a. general practitioners
   b. community nurses
   c. health visitors
   d. social workers
   e. community psychiatric nurses
   f. community clinics
   g. hospital accident and emergency departments
   h. chiropodists
   i. dieticians
   j physiotherapists

k. occupational therapists
l. speech therapists

(3) Secondary specialist services. Such services are based on large populations where the department of geriatric medicine forms part of the district general hospital. Patients with special problems are referred to them to sort out and manage complex matters which may then be referred back to the primary care professionals. This movement across the interface is important and has to be planned carefully.

The advantages of a generalist

Generalists are important, not merely as clinicians, but as a kind of ombudsman for the elderly patients with problems compounded of physical, mental and social elements. Their notes, well kept, and spanning many years, are unique documents and should match or outdo the memory of the patient.

The aim of the generalist is primarily concerned with the quality and standard of life of old patients. He will know the family, ethnic group, educational standard, and the hopes and aspirations of patients. He will understand and evaluate the effects on individuals, not only of pain and disability, but past occupation, retirement, bereavement, and relationships with other family members and neighbours.

He can establish a doctor/patient relationship based on continuity of care, rather than on intervention, so that his familiar presence is a source of comfort and reassurance to those who may have become isolated by age within their neighbourhoods.

The generalist is able to choose the right avenue for referral, and to communicate to the receiving officer the information he will need, but which the patient may not be able to supply. This will include psychosocial problems and modes of behaviour, as well as the use of aids and gadgets by the patient, and what might be needed in future.

He is best able to describe changes in behaviour which may be the first manifestation of disease processes likely to occur in old age, and the effects of these behavioural changes on family relationships. He may also note the consequences of awareness of deterioration in sociability, motivation, mood and sexual function. Above all, it is he who will note the interplay between the previous personality and experience of the patient and the present tendency to disengagement.

The doctor as the leader of the team

The concept of team care arose from geriatric practice, so it is reasonable to assume that one with a poor commitment to the care of the elderly should adopt a low profile in the team.

Leadership develops from authority and drive, which means that the member whose training is most demanded in a situation will 'lead' the team towards a solution. Thus, where there is a housing problem, the leadership would be expected to pass to the social worker. However, it is the general practitioner who is the longest serving member of most teams, and, were it not for his list of patients, there would be no attachments. He is the one who shoulders final responsibility for adequate patient care, and this places on him the managerial role of planning policy, organizing a service, communicating and delegating.

There is, however, the obvious need for all team members to agree on common policies, and, where decisions are to be made, the elderly people concerned should become *ad hoc* team members in decision making. Otherwise, much time may be wasted should they refuse what the rest of the team has decided for them!

Where to care?

There is little doubt that this should be in the home whenever possible. The hospital at home concept has worked well in other countries, when services, including intravenous therapy and specialist visits, are arranged by a social worker. It is surprising how much can be achieved by a well-organized team with experience.

Where this is not possible, there is everything to be said for the general practitioner caring for his patient in a community hospital. Unfortunately, these facilities exist only in certain districts. It is desirable for the beds to form part of the consultant's bed allocation, so that he pays a routine visit and can be called into consultation when needed.

WHAT DOES THE PATIENT WANT?

There is probably no more intimate doctor/patient relationship than with the elderly. A doctor will allow an elderly person of the opposite sex to embrace him as an expression of gratitude which he would avoid with a younger patient. He may hear death bed confessions of misdemeanours committed years ago, and ease the patient's passing by allowing this final ventilation. I have had a patient on the brink of death survive the week-end so that she could ask me on Monday morning to be sure to take care of her husband when she had gone, and then to see her sigh and the face go blanched as the sign of a death now permitted to happen.

Old people do not seem to want much. To younger people, they seem to wish for too little. That is because the confines of life have narrowed with a full realization of our human frailty. Nevertheless, for this very reason perhaps, we pay particular attention to the wishes of old people when they are expressed. Few appear to wish their lives to be prolonged, and treatments should be withheld if they are merely producing the extension of misery. In this respect, it is interesting that, in the first edition of Osler's famous textbook of medicine, he described pneumonia as the old person's 'enemy'. By the third edition, this had been changed to the old person's 'friend'.

Wishes that are not usually expressed are to have a caring doctor, on whom they can rely to relieve pain, especially the discomforts when dying, and to be present. Many patients will welcome the chance to talk about dying, the one certain event they still have to face. It can often be picked up as a subject from what appears to be random talk, such as: 'That was a bad heart attack. I thought I was going to die ......' This would allow a discussion to take place.

THE DYING PATIENT

It is a paradox that there is no event when attention to the needs of the whole person is more demanded than at the termination of a patient's life. We do not intend to discuss the medical aspects here, for they are covered at great lengths in other texts.

The patient who dies at home is almost always elderly. The care of the dying has replaced the gap left by domiciliary midwifery in the management of a great normal biological episode as a family doctor, rather than a technocrat.

To fulfil his role, the GP has merely to be present on a number of occasions, not just for his own persona, but as a representative of the larger profession he serves. Such matters cannot be taught – only experienced.

Of course, he assesses needs, mobilizes other team members, some of whom are more intimately involved in handling the patient. What he supplies is something else, quite apart from speech or drugs. By coming to see his patient, he may relieve anxiety, and support other members of the family. But most important, he fulfils a pseudospiritual role (if that is a meaningful term) by, in some way, conveying to the dying patient that he has not lived his life in vain. He would expect the presence of relatives, whose motives for gathering are various. The doctor, particularly if he is not involved now in medical care, indicates his value for his patient's life most dynamically when he cannot save it. This is often the apogee in the doctor/patient relationship, and it borders on closely to the role of a minister of religion, but should never encroach upon it.

Index

abdominal flank pigmentation 121
acanthosis nigricans 89,121
acoustic neuroma 101
affective disorders 151–8
ageing 58–81
   autoantibodies 68
   biology 61–3
   cellular level 60–1
   epidemiology 58–9
   exercise effect 77–8
   eye changes 69
   functional changes 70–1
   genetic aspects 59
   hearing changes 69–70
   immune response 68
   intrinsic theories 68
   physiological function 61–3
   psychological aspects 71–4
   sight changes 97–8
   stress 80–1
   understanding of speech 69–70
alcoholic neuropathy 150
alimentary system disorders 141–3
Alzheimer's disease 159, 162
amitriptyline 158
amnestic difficulties 26
amyloidosis 87
anaemia 148–9
   aplastic 149
   chronic lymphocytic 149
   iron deficiency 148–9
   megaloblastic 149
angina 111 (table), 135–6
angiotensin-converting enzyme inhibitors 106
anorexia 84, 85 (table)
anorexia nervosa 63
anticoagulants 137
anxiety 155–7
   management 157
aortic valve disease 136

aphakic eye 99
Argyll Robertson pupil 118
arrhythmia 136
arterial disease, peripheral 137
Asian communities 175–6
atrial fibrillation 136
at risk groups 166–70
   living alone 166–8
   retirement 169
attitudes in the care of the elderly 24
atypical presentation of diseases 21
Automated Geriatric Examination for
   Computer Assisted Toxonomy 163

back pain 110–13
bendrofluazide 109
benign senescent forgetfulness of Kral 71
bereavement 153, 173–4
beta-blocking agents 108
beta-lipoprotein 66
Betz cells 60
biguanides 147
biochemical indices 53
blood pressure 107–8
bone disorders 144–5
bowel function alteration 121
bronchial carcinoma 103
bronchitis, chronic 102

caffeinism 156
calcium antagonists 109
captopril 106, 109
carbenoxalone 180
carcinomatous neuropathy 151
cardiac surgery 135
cardiovascular disease 134–7
   prevention 134
Caribbeans 175
cataract 99
catastrophic reaction 73
causes of death 6

cerebrovascular disease 137–8
cervical spondylosis 96, 151
chest pain 109–10
children
   conflicts with 153–4
   divorce of 154
cholesterol, blood 66
claudication of cauda equina 110
Clifton Assessment Procedure for the Elderly 162
clinics 189–90
   assessment 189–90
   community 191
   special groups 190
confusion, acute 126–7
cor pulmonale 103, 136
country life 23
crisis intervention 186, 189
cultural aspects 174–5

day centre 191
day hospital 188
dementia 159–63
   definition 161–2
   language function 161
   language impairment 160
   management 162
   mental testing 160–1
   multi-infarct 162
dental hygiene 141
depression 81, 152–3, 157–8
   management 158
   unipolar 158
dexamethasone suppression tests 153
diabetes mellitus 146–7
   neuropathy 151
   visual impairment 98
diazepam 157
digitalis 106, 136
digoxin 181
diseases, insidious onset of 22
dissecting aneurysm 111 (table)
diuretics 106, 109
diverticular disease 143
dizzy turns 94–5
doctor
   generalist 196
   leader of team 197
   personal 55–6
   role 39
dorsal root pain 111
dothiepin 158
doxepin 158
drugs 182–6
   clarity of instructions 184
   combinations 184
   containers 184
   factors affecting action on elderly 182–3
   prescribing deadlines 183–4
   tablets 184
   unwanted effects 184
dying patient 198–9
dysphagia 85
dyspnoea on exertion 102–5
   cardiovascular causes 103–4
   congestive heart failure 104
   diagnosis 105
   management 105–6
   pulmonary causes 102–3

education 18–19
elderly *see* old person
emotional problems 153–4
emphysema 103
enalapril 106, 109
energy 64–9
   loss 89–90
ethnic groups 19
examination of patient 40–50
   alimentary system 49
   chest 46–7
   ears 42–3
   eyes 41–2
   heart 47–8
   lower limb 43–5
   neck 48
   rectum 49
   special senses 40–3
   spine 45–6
   upper limb 43–5
exercise 77–8
expectation of life 4 (table, 51 (figs.)

faecal impaction 49, 143
falls 22, 95–7

family 17–18
  future 18
family business 18
fatigue 89–90
fat shunt 66
feet 163–4
fenbufen 143
fire hazards 181
follow-up 56
free fatty acids 65
function state borderline 21

gallstones 142
general adaptation syndrome 80
generalist 196
Geriatric Mental State Examination 163
giant cell arteritis 98
glaucoma 99–100
glucocorticoids 66
glucose 65, 66, 75
  intolerance 66
gout 144
grandparenthood 17
growth hormone (GH) 65

haematological indices 53
Hayflick limit 60, 68
headache 93
health care, low expectations 20
health education 56
health visitor 35–6
hearing
  communication difficulties 26
  loss 100–2
hearing aid 42–3, 102
heat, effect of 22, 130
heavy–chain disease 149
herpes zoster 110, 150–1
  post–herpetic neuralgia 150–1
hiatus hernia 110, 111 (table), 142
high-dependency care 187–8
high-rise dwellers 23
Hindu women 176
hip pain 113–14
history taking 39–40
Home Help Service 191
hospital
  community resource 187–8
  day 189
  use of 187–8
hospital admission 54–5
  alternatives 55
  doctor's letter 54
  social problem effects 38
hospital investigations 188
hospital referrals 13–15, 188
housing 178–80
hydralazine 109
hypercapnia 103
hyperinsulinaemia 66
hypertension
  pulmonary 103
  treatment 108–9
hyperthermia 22, 130
hyperthyroidism (thyrotoxicosis) 118, 145, 156
hypochonadriasis 154
hypotension, postural 109
hypothalamus 63, 64 (fig.) 67
hypothermia 127–30
  management 130
  predisposing factors 129
  prognosis 130
hypothyroidism 145–6

iceberg effect 28, 29 (fig.)
imipramine 157, 158
incontinence, faecal 143
incontinence, urinary 122–6
  drug treatment 125
  follow-up 125–6
  home visit 123
  management 124
  referral 124
infective endocarditis 22, 136
influenza vaccination 136
inner city 23
insomnia see sleep disorders
institutionalization 176–7
insulin 65
insulinaemia 66
intellectual failure see dementia
intervertegral disc prolapse 112
investigations 50–3
  interpretation of test results 51–3
  normal laboratory values 53

ischaemic colitis 121, 143
isolation 72

jaundice 142
joint disorders 143–4
joint stiffness 77–8

Korsakoff's psychosis 150

laboratory values 21–53
laxative abuse 143
Leriche's syndrome 112
LH–FSH ratio 67
life span, effects of environment/life pattern 74
light-chain disease 149
living alone 167–8
locomotor system 143–5
long-standing illness, by age/sex 7 (fig.)
Looser's zones 144
low back pain 112

macular degeneration 100
malabsorption 142
male reproductive system, age-associated change 67–8
marital problems 153
memory impairment, short-term 73
menopause 63, 67, 68
  smoking effect 79
Marital Status Examination 160
metformin 147
methyldopa 109
Mobile Meals Service 191
monoclonal gammopathies (plasma cell dyscrasias) 149
morphine 136
motor neurone disease 150
multi-infarct dementia 162
multiple myeloma 112, 149
multiple pathology 21, 62–3
multiple sclerosis 118
muscle disorders 145
Muslims 175
myeloproliferative disorders 149
myocardial infarction 110, 111 (table), 135

naproxen 143
neuralgia, post-herpetic 151
neurodermatitis, nuchal 115
neurosyphilis 118
new town 23
nifedipine 109
nitrazepam 182
nurses 35
nutritional problems 84–9

obesity 74 (fig.), 75–7
  management 147–8
oedema, lower limbs 116–17
oesophagitis 142
oesophagus 142
  benign stricture 142
old people
  aims of care 194–5
  chronic conditions 8–11
  morbidity 8
  needs 197–8
  numbers in practice 6–7
  patient consulting doctor 10–11 (table)
  people providing care 195–7
Opren 184
osteoarthritis 144
  hip 113
osteomalacia 112, 144–5
osteoporosis 112, 144
  women smokers 79, 144
osteosarcoma 113

pacemaker implantation 136
Paget's disease 111, 112, 113, 145
  neurological disorders 151
pancreatic carcinoma 121
paracetamol 182
parent–child relationship 17
Parkinson's disease 117, 150
partial truths 24–6
past occupation 18
penicillin 181
peptic ulcer 142
phenytoin 180
phlebitis 137
pituitary gland 64 (fig.)
plantar response anomalies 44 (fig.)

plasma cell dyscrasias (monoclonal gammopathies) 149
pneumonia 139–40
  antibiotic therapy 141 (table)
  microbiology 140
  supportive measures 140
pneumothorax, spontaneous 103
polymyalgia rheumatica 145
polypharmacy 21
population, world 2–6
postural hypotension 109
practice organization 27–32
Pre-retirement Association 170
preventive care 27–8
prostate gland 49
pulmonary emboli 103, 137
pulmonary hypertension 103

receptionist 35
referrals to consultant 13, 54
reflux oesophagitis 110
reproductive homeostats 67–9
respiratory depressants 136
respiratory disease 138–40
retirement 169, 171–2
  preparation for 173
rheumatoid arthritis 143
roles in care of elderly 35–8

screening 28–32
  for/against 32
  record care 29, 30 (figs.)
self care 195
self-reporting of illness 20
senile traits 71
sex differences 17
sex problems 119–21
shakiness 117–19
sibling relationships 17
sick sinus syndrome 136
sight
  age changes 97–8
  communication difficulties 26
  extraocular causes of impairment 98–9
  macular degeneration 100
  ocular causes of impairment 98–100
  vascular occlusion 100
skin

excretory problems 181
  irritation 114–15
  delusional 115
sleep
  attitudes 90–1
  disorders 90–2
  causes 91
  drugs 91–2
smoking 79–80
social class factor 16
social problems 15–16
social workers 36
speech difficulties 27
spider naevi 89, 121
spouse 17–18
steatorrhoea 87
stress 80–1
Stroke Club 189
subacute combined degeneration (vitamin B_{12} deficiency) 151
sulphonylureas 147
suppurative parotitis 141
surface anatomy alteration 20–1
surveillance 189–90

T–cells 68
team 34–8, 185–6
  as a whole 185–7
  division of labour 36–8
testosterone, blood 67
tetracyclic antidepressants 158
thiazides 109
third party reports 20
thyrotoxicosis (hyperthyroidism) 22, 118, 145, 156
tremor 117–19
  cerebellar disease 118
  chronic alcoholism 118
  drug-induced 118
  emotional 118
  flapping 118
  multiple sclerosis 118
  neurosyphilis 118
  senile 118
  thyrotoxicosis 118
tricyclic antidepressants 157, 158
trigeminal neuralgia 150
triglyceride 66, 75

ulcerative colitis 143
unexpected recovery 22
unsteadiness 94–5

valvular disease 136
varicose veins 136–7
verapamil 109
vertebrobasilar insufficiency 94–5
vertigo 94–5
vision *see* sight
vitamin B_{12} deficiency (subacute combined degeneration) 151
volunteers 190–1

Waldenström's macroglobinaemia 149

weight loss 86–9
   diminished appetite/inadequate nutritional income 88
   examination 88
   good appetite/inadequate nutritional intake 87–8
   history 86
   investigation 88–9
   normal appetite/adequate nutritional intake 86–7
Weyrock system 191
whole person 194–8
widowed man 167
widowhood 153